Teaching Children *with* Pragmatic Difficulties *of* Communication

CLASSROOM APPROACHES

Edited by
Gilbert MacKay and Carolyn Anderson

Routledge
Taylor & Francis Group
LONDON AND NEW YORK

First published in 2000 by David Fulton Publishers

This edition published 2012 by Routledge
2 Park Square, Milton Park, Abingdon, Oxfordshire OX14 4RN
711 Third Avenue, New York, NY 10017, USA

First issued in hardback 2017

Routledge is an imprint of the Taylor & Francis Group, an informa business

British Library Cataloguing in Publication Data
A catalogue record for this book is available from the British Library.

ISBN 13: 978-1-138-16691-2 (hbk)
ISBN 13: 978-1-85346-650-2 (pbk)

Typeset by Elite Typesetting Techniques, Eastleigh, Hampshire

Contents

Notes on contributors

Carolyn Anderson is a lecturer in speech and language therapy at the University of Strathclyde, and also practises as a speech and language therapist in Renfrewshire and Inverclyde Primary Care NHS Trust.

Kirsty Gilbert is clinical specialist speech and language therapist in the Speech and Language Therapy Service of the Renfrewshire and Inverclyde Primary Care NHS Trust.

Roberta Lees is head of the Department of Speech and Language Therapy at the University of Strathclyde.

Jennifer Lundie is assistant head teacher in Chatelherault Primary School, Hamilton, South Lanarkshire Council, where she is in charge of the Autistic Spectrum Base.

Gilbert MacKay is research coordinator in the Faculty of Education, University of Strathclyde where he is also reader in special education.

Libby Roberts teaches art at Hollybrook Secondary School in the City of Glasgow Council.

All contributors are members of the team who teach the communication modules of the Support for Learning Diploma at the University of Strathclyde in Glasgow.

Acknowledgements

We should like to acknowledge gratefully the help the following colleagues gave us in preparing this book: Kellie Bracegirdle, Louise Brodie, Susan Brown, Jo Catterson, Lisa Glashan, Mary Horn, Heather Mackay, Marion McLarty, Elaine Porch, Anne Rooney, Adrienne Shaw, Stuart Ralston, Nan Wilson.

CHAPTER ONE

Useful communication

Gilbert MacKay and Carolyn Anderson

Background

In everyday life, 'pragmatic' means 'useful', 'functional' or 'what's right for just now'. In communication, it means just the same. 'Pragmatics refers to the use of language to express one's intentions and get things done in the world' (Gleason 1985, p. 22). This book has been written for teachers and speech and language therapists (SLTs) working in services for children who have difficulty communicating usefully. The range of literature dealing with their pragmatic difficulties is vast and sometimes inaccessible. We wanted to give fellow professionals a new guide to the topic, to help them take confident decisions about their daily practice. We want children with pragmatic difficulties to express their intentions and, as Gleason said, get things done in the world. But, first, we should say what we mean by pragmatic difficulties. Here are three examples. In each case and throughout the book, names and other identifying details have been changed.

Andrew

Imagine a service for children who have marked difficulty communicating. Its staff have built up a good relationship with the families of the children who attend, and have encouraged some to act as voluntary classroom assistants. Among these is the grandmother of one of the girl pupils. She is trying to help 9-year-old Andrew with a language puzzle on a computer program, but she is having some problems with the technology. Andrew turns to her and says in a calm, bland tone, 'You're a stupid old woman who never went to school anyway.' Surprisingly, she does not take offence. She has encountered pragmatic communicative difficulties before.

Brenda

Brenda is discussing a garden scene with her speech and language therapist. At 11, she is aware that she often knows what she wants to say but has problems finding the right words. She describes the insects she can see in the picture, 'There's a bee and a (long pause), a peanut butter.' 'Nearly,' prompts the therapist, 'It's a butter...' 'Fly.' says Brenda. The therapist asks Brenda what she can see growing under the ground. Brenda names them as globes. They are flower bulbs.

Colin

In class discussions, Colin rarely contributes. When meeting people, especially for the first time, he does not look at them but stares at his feet and shuffles continually. He gives the impression that he would rather be doing anything else than talking. Having a conversation with Colin can take a long time because his stammering speech makes it difficult to follow what he is saying.

Andrew, Brenda and Colin have pragmatic difficulties because they have problems communicating effectively. Yet, it is clear that these are three unique individuals with three quite different types of problem. Andrew's social gaffe is typical of the pragmatic difficulty that is seen in autistic behaviour. Brenda routinely has problems with double-meaning words and idiomatic phrases, which can be a frustrating barrier when she, her teacher and her fellow pupils do not take account of them. In school, Colin has no difficulty keeping up with the rest of his age group in lessons, and participates fully and equally as an ordinary member of his class. The examples were chosen for their diversity, but all of that diversity fits within a general context which is worth outlining in a little detail.

Pragmatics in principle – broad and narrow perspectives

From a historical perspective, pragmatics is the most recent of the language areas to be studied. The sciences of semantics (meaning) and syntax (grammar and word-ending rules) developed earlier and, in some ways, lent themselves more easily to objective study. Pragmatics tends to be less well known as it is a more recent research field, and as it has also suffered from a lack of commonly-accepted theory. Different researchers have generated different types of research depending on which view of pragmatics they take. In addition, each different way of understanding pragmatics may affect the type of intervention which is followed when working with people who have pragmatic difficulties. For this reason, it is important to know the current two main models of how pragmatics relates to linguistics – the other areas of language. Craig (1983) described relationships between linguistic and pragmatic rules in terms of either a narrow view of pragmatics or a broad view.

The narrow view treats pragmatics as one component in the language puzzle – it is as important as semantics and syntax but is independent from them. The practical implication of this perspective is that each component can be taught separately so that, for example, grammatical rules could be practised and learned without regard to their use in conversation. This view has perhaps been more prevalent among those speech and language therapists and linguists who use a 'deficit' model of intervention, targeting the more obvious surface features of difficulties. For example, this approach might involve intervention to help the development of syntax alone, with little emphasis on the underlying motivation for its use.

By contrast, the broad view of pragmatics is interactionist. Communication is seen as an integrated system of rules – pragmatic functions drive the choice of the elements of semantics and syntax. (See Bates and MacWhinney 1979, for further reading on this view; it is also discussed in Prutting and Kirchner 1987.) Each element of communication can be identified and studied but, in practice, it is only possible to understand semantics and syntax in relation to their achieving a desired purpose in communication. This point is important in reminding us that communicative purposes are the motivation for acquiring language in early development. Children learn the linguistic rules of their society which will help them achieve various goals through communication. Working in this model of pragmatics, intervention would use more natural social situations where communication functions provide the aims for using different linguistic codes. Teachers work from an educational model which places language in social context. They should have fewer problems accepting the interactionist model than therapists whose background in medical and linguistic models may, until recently, have inclined them to see difficulties in the area of pragmatics as distinct from those in the other areas.

Focus of the book

If language is like a puzzle, the 'narrow' view of pragmatics would treat the component parts as an inset board puzzle with a designated place for each. The 'broad', interactionist view would look at them like a Rubik cube. The interactionist view is adopted in this book. It may be complex and a little untidy at times, but that is the nature of communication too. Respect for that complex system influenced our choice of issues which the book should cover.

Chapter Two concerns the roots of pragmatic communication in early childhood. It shows how they make communication work by processes of action and interaction. Communication is action because it is an activity, and because it has a purpose. It is interaction because its success often depends on how well we relate to others. Making sense of difficulties in action and interaction is a challenge. The difficulties are varied and individualistic. There is a bewildering range of schemes that attempts to classify them. Chapter Two suggests that teachers and therapists might think of communication as a system. Other chapters refer to this systems approach, showing its potential in everyday work with children.

Pragmatic difficulties are outlined in Chapter Three. The discussion of communication as a dance, which was introduced in Chapter Two, is extended to group pragmatic skills into four main areas. The model of pragmatics as a dance sequence is intended to capture the integrated nature of communication and to connect behaviours which may appear unrelated. This framework is used to show which areas are likely to be most affected in children with different types of pragmatic difficulties.

Chapters Four and Five deal with the communicative difficulties of primary school pupils. In Chapter Four, detailed case studies are presented which describe the communication worlds of two children. The social and educational implications are discussed with recognition of the necessity for collaborative working to address each individual's very different needs. Chapter Five looks at case material on the pragmatic difficulties of a larger number of pupils in terms of the functions their communication can fulfil. It also gives details of a variety of strategies which teachers and SLTs have devised to make it more purposeful.

The book ends with three chapters dealing with how various systems may be organised to support pupils with pragmatic difficulties, their families and their professional helpers. Chapter Six deals with children who stammer. Conventionally, stammering is not thought of as a pragmatic difficulty but in a very real sense, it is. People who stammer have problems with making communication purposeful because of their difficulties in getting their ideas across. They have difficulties in the interactional aspects of pragmatics too, because of the disruption to normal rules of social interaction which is experienced by people who meet them. Chapter Seven deals with the system of the school. In particular, it shows how a school learned to respond to the educational and personal needs of a secondary school pupil with severe pragmatic difficulties through the medium of an action-research project. Finally, Chapter Eight reviews various dimensions of support that have to be taken into account if a service is to function well. Pragmatic communication is concerned with useful actions and interactions in the broad community. It is a complex task to set up structures that allow a system of support to operate there. This chapter gives guidance on aspects of provision, management and administration that enable this to be done more effectively.

Checkpoints

'Checkpoints' appear at various points throughout the book. Their purpose is to consolidate the points of what has just been read, and to help readers to relate the ideas to their own circumstances. These checkpoints are also designed to be points of focus for staff-development exercises in schools and special services, in which teachers and SLTs work together. They invite readers to go beyond the book into their own places of work and to relate its ideas to these settings. In that way, the processes of innovation and reflective practice give professionals and pupils new opportunities for useful – pragmatic – communication.

CHAPTER TWO

Actions and interactions: the roots of pragmatic communication

Gilbert MacKay

Introduction

Communication is sharing ideas. From birth, we behave as if the behaviour of other people towards us is intentional and purposeful – an attempt to let us share their ideas. We look for meaning in the acts of others, and we try to help them find meaning in ours. Sometimes our attempts to find meaning and to convey meaning are unsuccessful. Critical aspects of the activity's performance may be misleading, confusing, unusual or absent. For example, a reprimand from someone who is smiling might give a mixed message to any of us. Also, we may not use communication for a full range of its possible purposes. For example, some people may have difficulty using communication to share their feelings or to extend their knowledge and understanding. This can cause problems with relationships and with learning.

These examples are taken from two different aspects of pragmatics – the study of what communication achieves for us. The first aspect concerns relationships – how appropriate to their communicative partners are the forms of speech, writing, gesture or other behaviour which people use in acts of communication? The second aspect concerns purpose – how effective are acts of communication for achieving what people wish to achieve? There are many ways of trying to make sense of pragmatics in communication, but these two areas recur in different guises throughout a vast literature, and will form the basis of this chapter.

There is a detailed discussion of this two-sided view of pragmatics in sources such as van Dijk (1977) and Bachman (1990). Here, we shall look at how relationships and purpose develop in children's activity from their earliest days. Knowledge of this development gives insight into pragmatic difficulties which may cause concern in the school years and beyond. It should give teachers and therapists a clearer picture of how they may help children's communication to become more useful – more pragmatic, in fact. The next section of the chapter discusses the development of relationships in communication. Difficulties with the relationships that form and reform in acts of communication are probably the most striking evidence of pragmatic problems. After that, the chapter will outline the purposes which communication achieves, as these too have practical implications for work with children. The final sections of the chapter deal with attempts to find a useful framework for understanding pragmatics as a whole.

Why be concerned about frameworks? It is because practitioners often find it helpful to have points of reference that will enable them to understand their practice more quickly and accurately, so that they may make better decisions when faced with new challenges. Several examples of existing frameworks will be outlined, followed by a proposal for looking at pragmatic communication in a new and less complex way. Throughout the chapter, readers will be asked to stop to examine their own practice in the light of the issues that arise.

Relationships – the communication dance

This section of the chapter examines the interpersonal nature of communication. In particular, it examines it from a developmental point of view. The reason for this approach is that what appear as pragmatic difficulties in the school years and beyond, have parallels (if not their origins and roots) in early infant-adult interaction. The nature of this early interaction gives useful insight into later behaviours. Therapists and teachers can thereby see themselves as people who relate, rather than just as people who intervene. Difficult behaviour concerns them, but so do relationships.

The literature on early relationships in communication is more than 40 years old. Right from its start, that literature drew attention to the active part which both participants – usually infant and mother – play in developing their partnership. Stern (1977) says that this relationship is like a dance. There is a partner to whom we must relate, and a set of rules which gives formation to the relationship and the sequence of events in it. There is also an ebb and flow in intensity of movement, and sensitivity towards the individuality of one's partner, often with sharings that are unique to that relationship. Others can judge the quality of the dance because its rules are created, maintained and adjusted by a broader community. In competitive dancing, judges who are familiar with the culture give marks for the quality of precision of a performance – its closeness to a perfect execution of the rules. However, the individuality of the style of partnership is also given a mark. The partners in the relationship have rules within the rules which enable them to interpret the general principle according to their specific individuality. Precision and individual interpretation are important aspects of the dance of communication also.

That dance begins no later than birth, and may begin earlier. It has rules and conventions, and it recognises the presence of others. For over 20 years, it has been described and analysed by Colwyn Trevarthen, emeritus professor of psychology at the University of Edinburgh (e.g., Trevarthen 1977, 1988, 1993). Trevarthen has shown that, from birth, infants have an intellectual and communicative system that responds actively and emotionally to other people's presence and their attempts to communicate. Early interactions between mother and child help to direct the development of the child's thought, motives and emotions. They act to engage each other in a sustained relationship. Each responds to advances of the other as if they are expressing a similar set of feelings.

Thus, long before speech develops, infants converse with their mothers in 'protoconversations' which have the shared attention and other features of adult conversations – all that is missing are the words. In fact, it is not difficult to argue that the prototypes of words exist in these conversations, and not just in the 'parentese' (McTear and Conti-Ramsden 1992, p. 132) language of their parents. Trevarthen has noted that even the earliest contacts are concerned with cooperation, and with referring to events, topics and objects. Such referring prepares the ground for the appearance of symbols such as words. Their emergence becomes necessary as the child's range of experiences increases. They give a precision and efficiency that is not possible with the pointing, gesture and shared attention of early communicative behaviour.

Yet, in the context of this chapter, acquiring words is less vital than the inbuilt need to share meaning. Humans may well have a 'language acquisition device' (see, for example, Chomsky 1965). For practitioners, it is perhaps more important to think of the 'language teaching device' (Arkell 1986) which mothers demonstrate from the earliest days of their infants' lives. They are sensitive to the actions and reactions of the infants, and seem to move in time with them, as if to a rhythmic beat. Each behaves as if there is meaning and intent in their joint actions. This system is adjusted by both partners, so that contacts and relationships between each other are regulated. It is a partnership, with each influencing the other: the infants will be upset if their mothers' timings of reactions are not sensitive enough.

In early infancy, there are few references to events outside the interaction. This begins to change around six to seven months as the infants become aware of the effects of their own behaviour on others. Shyness, anxiety and showing off in the presence of strangers will be seen. People start to be characterised in terms of how familiar they are to the child. A little later, intimacy begins to emerge from this behaviour, and it can be thought of as the root of feelings of obligation towards others.

The early interactions have other features that seem connected both to efficient pragmatic communication and to pragmatic difficulties in later childhood. For instance, the mutual enjoyment of mother and child in these interactions leads them to establish rules for turn taking and overlapping in acts of communication. Subtle rhythms emerge. In later life, some children with pragmatic difficulties will have problems with these unwritten rules of engagement.

What is the purpose of this activity other than mutual enjoyment (not that there's anything unimportant about that)? Various aspects of cognitive, emotional and social development are involved, relating to children's needs, feelings, interests and purposes. Cognitive development will be dealt with in the next section of the chapter. Here, let us consider social and emotional aspects of communication that are connected with the area of pragmatic difficulties. For instance, infants' growing experience of other people – knowing who is familiar and who is not – helps them understand why others communicate, what their moods are, and what concerns them. They come to know what makes others tick and, in that process, become more individual persons themselves. In short, a great variety of social communicative activity occurs in the first year of life, and continues to develop thereafter. Here are some of its characteristic attributes.

- Butterworth (1998) describes the path towards the behaviour of pointing which begins when infants as young as two months follow, with their gaze, changes of direction in the gaze of adults. In turn, eye pointing gives the infants a powerful tool for controlling the behaviour of adults, by developing the *joint attention* of the partners in matters of interest to both of them.
- Joint attention relates to two other social aspects of communication, the *initiation* of communication, and the *maintenance of social interaction* for its own sake. The child and the adult work to build up rhythms of interaction (Hay and Demetriou 1998) – Stern's dance of communication, once more.
- A particularly important aspect of rhythm in communication is *turn taking*, poor sensitivity towards which may cause considerable problems in the pragmatics of communication (Ross and Goldman 1977; McTear and Conti-Ramsden 1992; Ninio and Snow 1996).
- Experience of relationships leads to *understanding of relationships* – in practice, knowing how to respond appropriately to a variety of people in a variety of settings. Appropriateness, or success, is evident when a harmonious communicative dance is maintained. That success will be one-sided, of course, when the needs of all participants in the activity are not met, or when one or more of the partners have not understood what was happening. This communicative skill is refined throughout life because we communicate in constantly-changing circumstances. All partners in communication have needs to be met by adjustment of the steps of the dance. That adjustment is not always successful.

Checkpoint 2.1

It's time to take a personal look at how children's early development of social skills through communication is relevant to people with pragmatic difficulties. Treat this as a two-stage workshop exercise with colleagues. The first stage is individual, concentrating on yourself. The second stage asks you to apply your insights to a child you know well.

Type of skill	*Success with skill*	*Difficulties with skill*
Joint attention		
Initiation of interaction		
Maintenance of interaction		
Turn taking		
Understanding of relationships		

Table 2.1 Early social-interaction skills

The left-hand column of the grid shown in Table 2.1 lists early social-interaction skills that have been mentioned in the section above.

- Make notes in the central column on when and how you yourself use these skills in communicating with other adults or with children.
- Then make notes in the right-hand column of any difficulties you yourself may have had in using the skills. Your notes will let you see that behaviour which begins to appear in early infancy, still has an important part to play in adult life.
- The second stage is a team effort. Identify a child with whom you and your colleagues work.
- Make notes in a fresh grid about the child. How well do they use the skills from infancy? When and how do they have difficulty with them?
- Now make notes on how you have responded to the child's needs, as they are affected by these difficulties. What strategies have been successful and unsuccessful? What new proposals would you, as a team, now make for the child?
- Make a list of priorities for action on the basis of the team's replies to these questions.

Purposes in early thoughts and actions

The focus on these social, interpersonal skills of communication is usually what is first thought of when practitioners mention pragmatic difficulties. However, pragmatic communication is concerned with more than the processes of interaction. Use the word 'pragmatic' with people in the street and they will think it relates to usefulness and serving purposes. Pragmatic has that meaning in the area of communication too. It is purposeful, useful or 'pragmatic' from the start. It helps us change and understand our world, and have an effect on the behaviour of other people.

This section, then, looks at the purposes of communication. What does it let us do? How does it affect other people? What is achieved by the social and interpersonal activity that was mentioned earlier? This aspect of pragmatic communication does not often appear in practitioners' publications on pragmatic difficulties: they generally concentrate on the social and interpersonal. However, the aspect of purposes does appear in texts for teachers, though it is rarely, if ever, described as pragmatic. Much of the language content of the National Curriculum (England and Wales), the 5–14 Curriculum (Scotland) and the Northern Ireland Curriculum is concerned with the development of these purposeful skills. For many years, they have also appeared in texts for professionals working with people who have intellectual impairments.

Action in communication

What, then are the purposes of communication? It is useful to begin answering that question from the standpoint of children's early development because it draws teachers' and therapists' attention to the range of dimensions that are evident from an early age if children are developing truly purposeful communication. Communication is sharing ideas. That proposal leads to questions about what we mean by ideas. I have suggested elsewhere (MacKay and Dunn 1989) that Piaget's classification of 'schemes' is particularly useful for identifying ideas that occur in the experience of young children. In addition, the classification can be a useful source of teaching activities when children begin to take an interest in the world, and start acting on it. In reality, the schemes are an amalgam of thoughts and actions which appear in the first 18 months of life (Piaget 1952, 1954; Uzgiris and Hunt 1975). They are outlined in Table 2.2.

The pragmatic thought-actions of the schemes become more sophisticated, and even change quite radically, as children grow, and begin to understand and use speech. However, it is worth spending a little longer on the purposes which they fulfil, for a number of writers have described pragmatic difficulties in ways that recall these early thought-actions. Lorna Wing illustrates them particularly well in describing the pragmatic difficulties of people with autism. The page numbers in the list below refer to her 1996 text.

Scheme	*Piagetian label*	*Explanation*
1	The development of visual pursuit and the permanence of objects.	Tracking moving objects; realising that an object continues to exist after it has disappeared from view; recognising familiar objects and people.
2	The development of means for obtaining desired environmental events.	Recognising own ability to change one's surroundings and meet one's needs.
3	The development of imitation: vocal and gestural.	(Self-explanatory)
4	The development of operational causality.	Recognising cause-effect relationships.
5	The construction of object relations in space.	Realising the importance of gravity, balance and the position of objects in relation to each other.
6	The development of schemes for relating to objects.	Manipulating and exploring the properties of objects and materials. The naming of objects is the highest point on this scale.

Table 2.2 The six sensorimotor schemes identified by Piaget

- *Object permanence* (scheme one) is concerned with distinguishing one object from another, recognising familiar things, not recognising things that are unfamiliar and knowing that out of sight is not out of mind – an object does not cease to exist just because we cannot see it. Wing comments on the reluctance of some children with autism to join in the classic object-permanence game of peep bo (Wing 1996, p. 34) and the even more fundamental activities of watching (p. 33) and taking an interest in the world (p. 34).

- It is possible that scheme two, *means-end behaviour,* is the most characteristically pragmatic thought action, for it is concerned with getting things done, and for being an active agent in that process. It was the scheme which Snyder (see Rees 1978) identified as the only distinguishing characteristic between children with normally-developing language, and those with delayed development. Wing (1996, p. 54) writes of the association between autistic behaviour and 'lack of motivation to engage in anything outside (one's) special interests'. Getting things done for oneself is low on the agenda of some people with autism, even at the level of expressing their needs to others.
- Problems with *imitation* (scheme three) can be seen both in some children's reluctance to join in cooperative games such as pat-a-cake (p. 34), and in the apparently unproductive ('echolalic') repetition of words and other vocalisations.
- With reference to *cause-effect behaviour* (scheme four), Wing notes that people with autistic behaviour may have 'an inability to put together all kinds of information derived from past memories and present events, to make sense of experiences, to predict what is likely to happen in the future and to make plans' (p. 25).
- Einstein famously drew attention to the close connection between the ideas of time and space. They are the subject of scheme five (*object relations*). There is much evidence for the connection of time and space in communication. For instance, words such as 'long', 'before' and so on, can relate to both time and space. As Wing shows (pp. 90–1), children with autism can have difficulty making sense of past and present experiences, and these may lead to special difficulties in understanding time and space.
- Children's *response to objects* (scheme six) has been used as a measure of their cognitive development. Children with pragmatic difficulties associated with autism may handle objects purely for physical sensations (p. 44) rather than in exploratory or functional ways. Professionals familiar with autism will often refer to other people being treated as objects rather than as beings. Treating people as objects can be useful developmentally, as can be seen in Trevarthen's and Hubley's (1978) discussion of 'person-person-object fluency'. However, problems can also arise when another person is engaged as a passive object rather than as someone who will make a response. For example (Wing 1996, p. 33): 'children with pragmatic communicative difficulties may not engage in the joint watching of events with their mothers that can lead to attracting the mothers' attention by pointing and making normal forms of eye contact.'

Checkpoint 2.2

Read through the bulleted list above. Think of a pupil or pupils with pragmatic difficulties in communication. Make notes on which, if any, of Piaget's six thought-actions are relevant to these difficulties.

Towards a pragmatic framework

It is reasonable to say, then, that knowing about the purposeful thought-actions of early childhood gives useful insight into pragmatic difficulties with communication. They can be a useful guide for working with children who have pragmatic difficulties, especially when combined with the interpersonal aspect of communication described in the earlier section of the chapter. However, there is a challenge in finding a useful framework that combines the purposeful and the interpersonal. Many attempts have been made, some to classify pragmatic behaviour, and some to be a basis for intervention. The complexity of the topic has made this task difficult. On the one hand, a framework must respect complexity if it is to be true to the nature of communication. On the other hand, it must be understood readily by busy practitioners if it is going to help them. Many existing approaches to classifying pragmatics do not do this. Some respect the complexity of pragmatics, but may be difficult to relate to everyday practice. Others may be accessible and useful, but not thorough enough in their cover of pragmatic communication. Still others may have a double disadvantage – not comprehensive enough, and difficult to understand! It is useful to look at some examples to discover what paths through a difficult territory are helpful.

Searle (1969) based an early classification scheme on the work of the Oxford philosopher, J. L. Austin (1962). He talked about pragmatics in terms of four kinds of 'speech acts', named 'illocutionary', 'perlocutionary', 'propositional' and 'utterance'. I have added these terms in brackets to the following brief, clear explanation of them by Prutting and Kirchner (1983, p.29):

> So, basically there is a speech act. The speaker means something (*illocutionary*), the sentence means something (*propositional*) and the hearer understands something (*perlocutionary*). In addition, there are basic rules governing the linguistic elements (*utterance*). These are the basic components ... of the speech act.

Searle's terminology is used widely in academic texts, but it is rarely talked about in school-based teams. Perhaps this is because it does not act as a helpful guide to description or intervention in such settings. Perhaps the language is just too off-putting. Yet, 'illocutionary' is a useful idea for practitioners working with people who have pragmatic difficulties. Think of it as meaning 'the purposes of communication' – describing, asking, demanding, socialising and so on. It encourages children to keep developing their speech and language. It is a step forward from the thought-actions of Piaget's schemes. It is also a focus on purpose which contrasts with the social and interpersonal aspects of pragmatics described by Trevarthen and the others who write about interactional behaviour.

Some schemes for classifying illocutionary purposes which have appeared over the years, are helpful when trying to understand and describe what goes on in language activities in classrooms and communication units. One of the most enduring is that of M. A. K. Halliday (1975), based on observations of the purposes of his young son's communication. It is outlined in Table 2.3 and put to practical use in Chapter Five.

Label	*Purpose*	*Example in adult language*
Instrumental	Satisfies speaker's needs	I want ...
Regulatory	Controls others	Do this
Interactional	Fosters relationships	Hello
Personal	Expresses own uniqueness	Here's what I think
Heuristic	Increases knowledge	Tell me why ...
Imaginative	Creates world of make-believe	Let's pretend ...
Informative	Recounts experiences	I've something to tell you

Table 2.3 Purposes of single-word utterances (MacKay and Dunn 1989, based on Halliday 1975)

It is a short step to the classroom from theoretical classifications of communicative purposes, such as that of Halliday. In the UK, Joan Tough (e.g., 1976, 1981) created an influential language-development approach based on the following 'illocutionaries':

- self-maintaining (by asserting one's own presence, and establishing relationships);
- directing (commands, orders and instructions);
- reporting on present and past experiences;
- towards logical reasoning;

- predicting (consequences);
- projecting (putting oneself in another's situation);
- imagining (creative thinking and fantasy).

Tough's approach to the teaching of language had a major impact on British preschool and primary education twenty years ago. It was never labelled a 'pragmatic' scheme by teachers or teacher educators, yet pragmatic it was. It proved to be a useful form of early intervention for developing young children's language skill in a range of purposes, aimed at helping them to learn and communicate more effectively.

It is important to see Tough's work in its historical context. She was writing at a time when there was a strong commitment to intervention in the linguistic development of children in the upper preschool age range and the early years of primary school. This intervention was intended to counter the effects of any factors in experience and upbringing that might be disadvantageous to the development of oral language. It assumed that focused intervention in children's development of oral skills would benefit their development of literacy and other scholastic activity. Special services and units were set up in various parts of the United Kingdom to respond to this perceived need. Some still exist, though their function may well have changed now, because of a more recent educational preoccupation with pragmatic difficulties. Increased attention to groups of children with difficulties of language, communication and autism arose on a widespread scale in the UK especially from the early 1990s, and this concern continues to grow.

Tough's work had a particularly powerful influence on British primary education and teacher education in the 1970s and 1980s, but hers was not the only well-known attempt to clarify pragmatics effectively. For example, Dore (1978) built a system on the acts of requesting, asserting, responding, regulating , expressing and performing. McShane (1980) created another around regulation, stating, exchanging, personal references and conversation. In 1994, Ninio *et al.* reviewed the field of pragmatic classifications exhaustively. (See also Ninio and Snow 1996.) The reason for their review was their belief that existing systems for classifying pragmatics:

- were limited in scope;
- did not cover the entire developmental range of people from birth, nor did they include people with disabilities as well as those with standard development;
- were limited in their theoretical foundations;
- had debatable empirical bases.

The review by Ninio *et al.* was a major contribution to the academic study of communicative acts. The extent of its applicability to educational and clinical practice is less clear. It is a complex system, with 12 categories and 67 subsections, and it was not designed to aid intervention. However, the researchers also offered a second framework of just six main classes of speech interchange. These are outlined in Table 2.4.

Class	*Explanation*
Negotiations	Directions to the listener, commitments by the speaker, declarations about a state of affairs
Markings	Communications to signal that an event has occurred
Discussions	Exchange of information in an established and sustained conversation
Performances	Carrying out verbal moves – rule-bound activities within an agreed and understood framework determined by the communicators and/or the social setting in which they live
Metacommunications	Demands for clarifications so that the hearer can understand the communication of the speaker (or writer) more clearly
Uninterpretables	The intent of the interchange is not clear

Table 2.4 Outline of the classes of speech interchange identified by Ninio *et al.* 1994

Ninio's team make strong arguments for the adoption of this framework in the study of pragmatic communication. What is more, it acts as a useful umbrella for the classification of the work of other writers mentioned in this chapter, in terms that are sometimes more lucid than those of the original work, as Table 2.5 shows.

Class (from Table 2.4)	*Related phenomena in other schemes*
Negotiations	Requestives, expressives, performatives (Dore 1978) Instrumental, regulatory, interactional, personal (Halliday 1975) Regulation, statement, exchange, personal (McShane 1980) Self-directing, other-directing, self-maintaining (Tough 1976) Communicative intentions (Dewart and Summers 1995)
Markings	Assertives (Dore 1978) Responses to communication (Dewart and Summers 1995)
Discussions	Responsives (Dore 1978) Informative (Halliday 1975) Statement, personal, conversation (McShane 1980) Reporting on past and present experiences (Tough 1976) Interaction and conversation (Dewart and Summers 1995)
Performances	Assertives, regulatives (Dore 1978) Regulatory, interactional, personal (Halliday 1975) Regulation, exchange, personal, conversation (McShane 1980) Empathetic, self-maintaining, interactional (Tough 1976) Interaction and conversation, response to communication, contextual variation (Dewart and Summers 1995)
Metacommunications	Requestives, expressives (Dore 1978) Heuristic, imaginative (Halliday 1975) Conversation (McShane 1980) Reasoning, predicting, imagining (Tough 1976)
Uninterpretables	...

Table 2.5 Relationships between the six pragmatic categories of Ninio *et al.* 1994 and previous attempts to classify pragmatic behaviour

> ### *Checkpoint 2.3*
>
> Existing frameworks for pragmatics are based primarily on the behaviour of people with few difficulties or none. You may or may not find that they are helpful for describing the pupils with whom you work. Look again at the frameworks in this section of the chapter to discover how useful they may be. Keep a particular pupil (or group of pupils) in mind, and mark terms in Table 2.4 which are useful for drawing attention to their pragmatic difficulties.

Reflection on existing frameworks

The appeal to practitioners of the Ninio six-part classification lies in its grounding in evidence and argument, its relative simplicity and its honesty in including an 'uninterpretable' category. It is also a scheme that lends itself well to the description of nonverbal and preverbal communicative acts. In addition, it brings within a common frame of reference the two types of pragmatics covered by this chapter – action and interaction. Yet there are some gaps in translation which make it unlikely that this powerful descriptive system might also be a framework for teaching pupils with pragmatic difficulties. For instance, it is concerned mainly with the functions of communication and does not accommodate the problems with understanding which many people with pragmatic difficulties experience. Examples can be found throughout the chapters of this book. Also, the framework does not need to take particular account of context: its function is to describe acts of communication, rather than to make sense of difficulties in making these acts effective.

The very thoroughness of the work that led to the proposals of Ninio *et al.* casts doubt on the worth of searching for a more elaborate classification system, at least in intervention settings such as schools and special services. Is there, then, a different way of understanding pragmatics that would be more applicable?

Systems

There is a useful, positive answer from systems research. It recognises that systems such as schools, clinics and companies are complex. Rarely will there be a simple way of understanding or evaluating them. They need to be understood in various different ways simultaneously. It is the same with communication – any normal conversation involves (among other things) vocabulary, grammar, speech inflections, interpersonal courtesies, purposes and so on. Thus, communication can be understood as a special type of system.

One powerful technique of systems analysis for examining schools has been proposed by Bela Banathy (1973, 1992, 1996), and has been developed by the author and colleagues (MacKay *et al.* 1996; McCartney *et al.* 1998). Banathy suggests that we should look at systems in terms of photographic ideas: the still picture, the moving picture and the bird's eye view:

- the still picture looks at *functions* and *structures*;
- the moving picture looks at *processes*;
- the bird's eye view surveys the overall influence of the *system* on its *environment*, and of the environment on it.

Table 2.6 sets these ideas in the context of acts of communication.

The final, and extended, checkpoint of the chapter asks you to bring the four rows of Table 2.6 into the context of your own individual needs for describing pupils' difficulties. That exercise may give hints for structuring reports for review meetings and other monitoring of children's progress. A good structure for reporting, of course, may well be a useful guide for intervention too.

Banathy's image	*Aspect of system*	*Meaning*	*Example of effective communication*	*Example of difficulty*
Still picture (1)	Function	What communication is meant to achieve	Asks for something to eat and receives it	Draws attention to oneself in a way that arouses others' indignation rather than empathy
Still picture (2)	Structure	The means by which communi-cation is achieved	Uses vocabulary and grammar that are understood easily	Uses a limited, stereotyped range of conversa-tional gambits
Moving picture	Process	The sequence of the act of communi-cation	Balances a conversation successfully between speaking and listening	Fluent, loquacious speech, but with little attention to the content of what the other partner is saying
Bird's-eye view	System-environ-ment interaction	How the act of communication takes account of surroundings and how it influences them	Converses successfully in a wide range of circumstances in in everyday life	Successful conversa-tions occur in a limited range, of familiar, predictable circumstances

Table 2.6 Understanding communication as a system in Banathy's (1992) terms

Checkpoint 2.4

Using the 'still picture'

The two parts of the still picture deal with functions and structures – respectively, what pupils use communication to do, and the means by which they achieve it. The 'functions' aspect considers the purposes which children's communication is achieving, or is not. The 'structures' aspect examines how the functions are able to occur, or are not. The 'still picture' is an area to which teachers and SLTs bring skills which sometimes overlap and which are sometimes different. This is a good basis for collaborative working.

The 'still picture' – functions

Look again at the notes you made on the Ninio framework at Checkpoint 2.3. Use them to identify the purposes for which your pupils do, or do not use communication successfully.

1. With a particular pupil (or group of pupils) in mind, list terms from your Table 2.4 notes which are useful for pinpointing their pragmatic difficulties.
2. Make a note of any difficulties which are not covered by the terms in Table 2.4. Suggest your own terms for these difficulties. For example, functions such as 'making friends' may be more important to a child of whom you are thinking than are some of the others mentioned.
3. Add 'other' to your list, to cover the unexpected.

The 'still picture' – structures

The list of possible structures that may be relevant to all children is complex to specify. Try to think of them as attributes, and ways of thinking, organising and working that let us carry out the functions of communication. They include:

- spoken vocabulary;
- grammatical constructions;
- understanding the meanings of words and phrases;
- being aware of intent in the communication of others;
- having flexible frames of reference, so that the right vocabulary, intonation, grammar, and so on are selected for the right occasions.

1. Select items from this list that suit your own pupil (or group of pupils) well.
2. Add to the list, or adapt it, in the light of your own experience and needs.
3. Add 'other' to your list.

You now have the beginnings of a memory aid for describing communication in action, in the individual circumstances of a child or children with whom you work. Treating the 'moving picture' and 'bird's-eye view' in a similar way, will complete that process.

The 'moving picture' – process

This 'moving picture' deals with communication in action. What do you learn about pupils' communicative strengths and needs by watching them try to communicate? The processes of communication include behaviour such as:

- taking turns in play or conversation;
- starting, maintaining and ending acts of communication appropriately;
- showing awareness of rules of exchange: for example, knowing how to respond when others communicate; knowing to stick to the theme of a conversation (though not rigidly!);
- coping with interruptions, problems and unexpected events that may arise in any act of communication.

Once again, draw up a list that meets your needs for describing the processes of communication that are particularly relevant to your pupils.

The bird's-eye view – system-environment interaction

The 'bird's-eye view' is concerned with how effectively pupils communicate in real life, outside the controlled settings that are created for them in classrooms and units. It considers how pupils are influenced by their surroundings, and especially by the people in them, when they communicate. It also considers what effect their communication has on these people. This is a wide-ranging view of the system of communication, taking account of real-life communication, and the services that exist to facilitate it.

- In how wide a range of circumstances do the pupils have opportunities to communicate? Is it controlled restrictively by professional workers and family? Or do they have the chance to learn in a variety of real-life settings by trial and error and trial and successful choice? What can be done to increase their opportunities for communicating in circumstances that are beyond the familiar and the controlled?
- In what real-life settings have the pupils shown that further skill is needed? Answering this question may give guidance on what to rehearse in the safe surroundings of home and school, so that later experiences have a better chance of success.

- To what extent do pupils recognise when they have difficulties understanding other people, and being understood by them? How do they cope with such experiences? What support do they need, so that their confidence and self-esteem are not harmed, both at school and in the real-life location where the communication occurs?
- What is the extent of interprofessional collaboration, so that all services concerned with the communication of the pupils are collaborating effectively? (This is a 'structure' question too.)
- What is the extent of home-school-service links?

Coda

Your own experience, in the form of your notes on functions, structures, processes and real-life relevance, will give you a useful tool for auditing the circumstances of children who have pragmatic difficulties in communication. This may be helpful in formulating plans of action for these children, by identifying strengths, needs and priorities for action. The later chapters of this book will take you further on the journey among actions and interactions, building on the experience of other practitioners who have addressed different aspects of that challenge.

CHAPTER THREE

Pragmatic communication difficulties

Carolyn Anderson

Introduction

This chapter covers the main pragmatic problems which can arise in communication, by comparing communication with a dance. The aim is to give pragmatic skills some structure and to make connections between what often seem to be unrelated behaviours. This diverse collection of difficulties such as eye contact, topic maintenance, facial expression and inference can often be difficult to understand. Thinking of communication as a dance suggests that different pragmatic areas are associated with different types of communicative activities and difficulties.

The pragmatic dance

Banathy (1992), referred to in Chapter Two, said that aims are the reason systems exist. Pragmatic aims are the various *functions* of communication which motivate us to interact – asking, sharing thoughts, describing and so on. These pragmatic functions are the music which allows the dance of communication to begin. Banathy also examined the *structures* which support the aims, and are the means by which the aims can be achieved. The structures of the communicative dance which let the functions be realised are pragmatic behaviours. These are used to signal different meanings in conversation by means which include turn taking, nonverbal expression and features in the flow and pitch of speech. These behaviours are the steps of the dance. Banathy's description of systems also included the matter of *process*. For the communication dance, the process is the pattern of the interaction of partners. Finally, Banathy's *systems-environment* relationship is the dance floor – the external context in which the dance takes place, which affects the dance, but which may also be affected by it. The context of communication includes matters such as culture, education and social relationships.

Making music

We communicate for a purpose, to express some meaning. This intention emerges in infancy and develops from nonverbal communication into conversations which are mainly verbal but continue to include many nonverbal elements. The underlying meanings or functions are what motivate us to communicate. They include making requests, demanding, or explaining. They are the music which makes the dance of communication necessary. The number of functions for which we can use communication are numerous and have been listed by authors such as Halliday (1985). Our main purpose in all these acts of communication is to get our meaning across and achieve the desired function.

So how is the meaning or 'music' understood? It may be helpful to digress briefly into language philosophy which tries to explain how we understand more than is actually said. Austin's speech act theory tried to explain how utterances are understood by distinguishing among:

- what is said;
- what the force or intended meaning is;
- the effect of this meaning on the hearer. (Austin 1962)

The speech act sets the utterance firmly within a situation in order to understand its meaning. In order to understand a sentence we need to know not only the grammatical structures used and the meaning of the words. We must also relate both of these understandings to the context in which it is used and to our world knowledge to make sense of it. For example, if you heard this sentence: 'He wound up with a real belter,' you would be able to recognise the grammatical construction and the vocabulary. You would also be able to think of possible social scenarios to which it might apply but its meaning in relation to you would be reduced if you did not have knowledge of the specific context. If you knew the person speaking was a keen music fan talking about a concert, your understanding of the sentence would be different from that of following a discussion about someone's eventual selection of a mate, or about a boxing match.

However, using context and understanding the utterance's literal meaning are not always sufficient to explain how we interpret what a speaker intends. As speakers, we use a combination of statements which are exactly what we mean, as well as statements with an implied meaning. For example, someone may say, 'Lovely weather' when it is raining. We understand the utterance's normal meaning but, given the context, the only way we may be able to make sense of this statement is to assume the speaker is being ironic. Grice (1981) says we do this by assuming that our conversational partner is cooperating in the conversation and is following four basic conventions in expressing meaning. These four conventions – Grice calls them 'maxims' – concern quantity, quality, relation and manner. The maxims state that:

- the amount of information given will be sufficient ('quantity');
- what is said will be relevant ('quality');
- what is said will be based on what you believe to be truthful ('relation');
- it will be both brief and clear (that is, not deliberately ambiguous or obscure).

The maxims help us to make sense of implied meaning. Sometimes we can imply meaning by using specific words like 'but', 'even', 'therefore', 'yet', 'for', as in the example of 'She's nice, for a teacher', or 'He's naughty but he means well.' We can also use the same words to imply different meanings in different conversational circumstances, so that 'Just what I always wanted' may imply genuine appreciation, disgust, exasperation, and so on. Having heard the statement, it is then up to the listener to infer what the implied meaning may be, using the assumptions of cooperation, the conversational maxims and knowledge of the context. (See Thomas 1995, for further discussion.)

Checkpoint 3.1

Think about some situations where the same words are used to perform different speech acts (for instance, 'I'll be back' could be used as a promise, a threat or a compliment). Now think about a situation where different words could be used to perform the same speech act (for instance, asking someone to move, because they are blocking your way).

Relevance theory (Sperber and Wilson 1995) states that only one maxim is needed to explain both implied and explicit meaning. It is that a speaker will make each communication as relevant as possible, taking into account the context and previous knowledge of the listener. The listener is able to infer the speaker's intended meaning, using both cognitive understanding and pragmatic comprehension. But communication becomes difficult if a speaker's intentions cannot be inferred. Literal information may be understood to some degree, but lack of inference will spoil understanding of subtle, high level interaction such as irony, metaphors and conversational subtext.

Another major area of interest in pragmatics is presupposition. It focuses on the assumptions underlying some words and on the presuppositions necessary for successful communication. Some verbs may carry assumptions such as 'I forgot that I had lost my umbrella', which lead the listener to presuppose that it is true that I did lose my umbrella. The ability to make these assumptions depends to a large degree on understanding another's point of view.

In conversation, we often use a shorthand method to refer to items in context, as we understand that our conversational partner is sharing the same information. For example, in 'This is Edward's book, can you pass it on to him?' the listener knows that 'it' refers to the book and 'him' refers to Edward. Similarly, 'Stand over there' is only meaningful for the listener in context, that is when the listener can see where the speaker is indicating. These expressions are dependent on context if we are to interpret them correctly, and are known as 'deixis' in the study of communication. The extent to which deixis pervades our language use is often apparent only when someone fails to use it. This results in stilted language and the impression of overformality.

Checkpoint 3.2

A six-year-old boy was labelled as a behaviour problem in the infant class because he did not obey instructions that his teacher gave to the class in general. His difficulty in making assumptions meant that when the teacher said 'Everyone, get out your books', he did not think she was talking to him but to a child called 'Everyone'. His 'disobedience' disappeared when she gave him instructions prefaced with his name. Can you think of a recent experience when you have made an erroneous assumption which has led to communication breakdown?

The steps of the dance

In Banathy's model the aims of a system are supported by structures. In the dance of communication, the structures are the steps or rules. Conversational rules help us to achieve the communication functions we have chosen. For communication to be successful, both partners should know the rules, just as in a dance both partners need to know the steps, to perform each type of dance. Many of these rules will be similar for different language aims, but some behaviours will be more appropriate to achieve an aim than others. Pragmatic competence reflects ability to make these adjustments. So, if the music is the foxtrot, steps or behaviours might be adjusted slightly compared with those for a waltz but the features would still be recognisable as 'dancing'. Pragmatic rules can be divided up into four main types of steps.

- Linguistic rules cover those steps which require the partners to give and receive meaning. Examples involving choices in both appropriate vocabulary and grammar are discussed above and outlined in more detail below.

- Rules for conversational flow govern procedures such as taking turns in conversation.
- Prosodic features determine how we use intonation, volume of speech, rate of speech, and so on.
- Nonverbal rules concern facial expression, eye contact and nearness to one's partner when communicating.

Linguistic behaviours let the speaker match grammar and vocabulary to the purpose of the communication. In normal language development, children begin with limited grammar and vocabulary choices but their parents use context to understand the underlying meaning. For example, when an 18-month-old child says, 'Sock', her parents may understand a variety of meanings from this word depending on the situation – naming the item, or a request to put the sock on, help find it, or remove it from the dog's mouth.

As children develop language skills, their choices in expression expand. But as the choice increases, so do problems of storing and retrieving language information. Vocabulary may not always be as accessible as expected, as we sometimes cannot remember the exact word we want to use. This problem is often associated with increasing age and failing memory, but it is a normal occurrence for speakers throughout life. The problem can be overcome by different methods such as using a similar word, describing the function of the item or action, or recalling the initial sound to help to jog the memory. Grammatical knowledge may be more robust but there may occasionally be problems with the order in which words are said, especially when forming more complex sentences.

The second type of pragmatic rules govern conversational flow. The main feature which facilitates this is that speakers and listeners take turns. To do this competently, turns must be coordinated. So, silences are short, and a smooth handover to the next speaker is achieved by using appropriate signals. These signals can be made with a number of prosodic and nonverbal features such as a drop in pitch or increased eye contact as a turn is ending. In Chapter Two, early interactions were discussed where child and parent took turns in preverbal conversation and used nonverbal signals. As language develops, turn taking depends not only on recognising these pragmatic behaviours but also on applying linguistic knowledge to predict more accurately when a speaker's turn will end. Turn taking in conversations can be problematic when partners refuse to give up their turn or when they fail to accept the handover of a turn. McTear and Conti-Ramsden (1992) have summarised many of the research studies in turn taking and overlaps.

The third set of pragmatic rules relate to prosodic features such as intonation, volume and speaking rate. For example, a sentence can be changed from a statement to a question by using a rising intonation pattern as opposed to a pitch drop as the sentence finishes. Intonation and elongating the final syllable of a word are important signals for turn taking which children learn to recognise and use.

Volume can be used to emphasise words to make a point, imply that information is confidential and so on. Rate of speech is often modified depending on the age or perceived understanding level of the listener. For example, adults tend to speak more slowly to children, people with hearing problems or non-native speakers of a language.

The fourth type of pragmatic conversational rules govern nonverbal behaviours such as facial expression, eye contact, gestures and proximity. These features along with prosodic signals are often how we communicate underlying emotional meaning such as sincerity, anger, joy or indifference. As discussed above, eye contact is important in coordinating conversational turns and it is also used to indicate interest and attention between partners. In normal conversations, listeners look at speakers more than speakers look at listeners. Facial expression is a powerful indication of emotional responses, hence the phrase, 'Your face speaks volumes.' Proximity between partners is largely determined culturally. Closer proximity usually implies a closer relationship, so that partners who violate these rules and invade personal space may make communication uncomfortable.

Just as dances may be simple or more intricate, obvious behaviours in communication may be used to signal intent as well as more subtle signs. For example, we may choose to use shorthand signals with a well-known partner who is familiar with their use because this is more efficient. An example discussed above is the use of pronouns in deixis. Facial expressions, intonation, and other pragmatic behaviours can also be interpreted in different ways depending on whether our partner is new or more familiar.

Partner interaction

A good dance sequence requires the partners to be coordinated and this is usually achieved through the dance steps described in the previous section. Just as in a dance, communication will tend to be more successful if partners are skilled at the steps or if they are familiar with each other. Skill also involves being able to retrieve the situation if a wrong step is made. Dancers have to be able to cope with fast as well as slow dances. They may also have to deal with interruptions and distractions. Improvisation is frequently the norm in the communication dance but changes in topic must be introduced as seamlessly as possible to ensure a successful performance. And finally, dancers need to be able to cope with 'reels', where multiple partners make the dance more complex. Discourse analysis is the method used to study the dance itself, and is the context for discussing each of these features, below.

Partners need to be coordinated in conversation so that they are ready to take their turn on the conversational floor when their partner has finished speaking. In conversation, coordination is achieved by following the rules and by giving feedback as listeners, to indicate to their partners that they are following the conversation. Feedback is usually given by eye contact, and also by various other encouraging behaviours such as nodding, verbal agreement like 'huh', and by mirroring the body posture of the speaker.

One partner may be more skilled than the other and may compensate for the less skilled partner. For this reason each partner's role in the interaction needs to be evaluated. As discussed in Chapter Two, parents initially fill in much of the 'missing' or verbal communication of their infants in protoconversations until the child gradually develops more communication skills. Problems may show with less skilled partners. For example, some children may prefer adult interaction and find peer interaction more difficult. This difficulty may be because adults are more adept at retrieving conversations when communication breakdown occurs.

Conversations may break down when a listener does not understand what a speaker has said. Listeners may or may not recognise that they have not understood. If they do recognise this, they must be able to signal that they need clarification. The speaker must then be able to repeat, rephrase or elaborate on the information to repair the breakdown. When partner interaction breaks down, children may fail to recognise that there is a problem. Making successful requests for clarification, and successful responses to them, depends on linguistic and pragmatic competence. Children with SLI or pragmatic difficulties are likely to have more conversational breakdowns and have fewer strategies with which to repair misunderstandings (McTear and Conti-Ramsden 1992).

The pace of conversation tends to be negotiated by partners as they speak, and may also be determined by factors in the situation of the conversation, such as time constraints or interruptions. Parents often automatically slow the pace of interaction for young children, to allow them time to process what is being said and to formulate a reply. In normal development, children learn to cope with a faster, adult pace of conversation. Some children will be able to cope with a slower pace of conversation, while a faster pace may expose more problems. A faster pace puts all language areas under pressure, while a slower pace allows more processing time. For this reason, even adults prefer a slower pace when listening to more complex topics and discussing them.

Conversational turns are not always accomplished smoothly, and so children learn to deal with interruptions and distractions in developing pragmatic competence. Interrupting a speaker is sometimes necessary to gain the conversational floor and can be used effectively in conversations. However, it often carries social implications, and requires confidence. Our knowledge of language can help in judging where the least disruptive point is for an interruption. As every parent knows, young children tend not to have developed this fine tuning in interrupting adult conversations, and must be taught the necessary social rules.

In conversation, exchanges between partners tend to have cohesion and coherence so that the discourse is connected. Speakers use links to establish cohesion at a linguistic level by techniques such as deixis – for example, using pronouns to refer to the person being discussed. To keep conversations coherent, partners share a topic and develop themes around it. Speakers signal to listeners if a conversational topic is going to change. Usually this is accomplished with an introductory phrase such as, 'By the way' or, 'Before I forget'. Without such a warning, a partner can be wrong footed as switching the tune or topic can lead to confusion.

Conversations with multiple partners are a more complex dance. Interaction in a group is more difficult because turn taking is less clearly defined, and so interruptions and overlapping turns are more likely to occur. Fewer opportunities may exist for repairing breakdowns satisfactorily for each participant, for requesting clarification or for controlling the conversational pace. Social rules may affect turn taking in groups. Any difficulties in group interaction may inhibit participation in this type of dance. That is why committees have formal procedures, such as deferring to the chair, to ensure that their processes are effective.

The dance floor

Communication takes place in an environment which includes elements such as social relationships, culture and education. These are its dance floor. Language and social skills are inextricably linked. For young children, one of the main motivations in using language is to engage another in play. For this reason, many parents note an increase in language use when a child enters nursery. During the early school years, children use language for many social functions such as entering their peer groups or negotiating rule setting in games. By adolescence, language becomes a means of exploring and establishing one's unique place in the world. Throughout this development, children become adept at using language with an increasing number and range of social partners, who may not be as accommodating as their parents. (See Gallagher 1991 for discussion of social language use.)

Cultural expectations affect pragmatic areas, such as who can start a conversation, as do the grammatical forms used between people of different social relations. Culture also determines a variety of nonverbal behaviours, such as eye contact, proximity, posture and facial expression, as well as prosodic features such as intonation and volume of speech. These elements are bound up with spoken language and are appropriate to the community in which they have developed. A different culture may have different expectations of what is appropriate. These rules for pragmatic interaction will be learned along with the spoken language.

Pragmatic rules are often subtle, and may not be initially obvious to the learners of a second language.

Educational expectations also affect communication, as the child learns to understand and use more formal language with teachers and adults outside the family. The social purpose of communication is stressed in educational contexts. It is important that children can learn to use a variety of communication forms in natural situations, for example, the different partner interactions which are required in the classroom, such as small group work, circle time and so on. (See Tough 1977 for approaches to communication functions which may be taught systematically in the classroom.)

Types of dancing problems

Pragmatic ability depends on developing both the understanding and social use of language. To do this, children must be able to learn about language rules and their social applications. Pragmatic difficulties are common where a child's cognitive understanding, language or social-emotional development is delayed or disordered. This section reviews some such difficulties in terms of a dance interrupted.

Problems in hearing the music

We have seen that meaning may be understood by combining linguistic understanding with contextual information and previous knowledge. Meaning is also based on the assumption that our communication partner is cooperating and working from a similar set of principles. Mistakes and misunderstandings may occur when we are deliberately misled, or if someone has difficulty in interpreting the message. Problems in understanding pragmatic meaning are normal. Most communicators will be able to recognise and repair misunderstandings. However, children with problems in pragmatic understanding will routinely fail to comprehend, or let people know that they have not understood the meaning.

In pragmatic development, joint attention must be established initially. This constitutes the motivation and agreement to dance. A child with difficulty in this area will have fewer opportunities for learning pragmatic routines. Pragmatic comprehension begins from an early age, when children interpret nonverbal cues such as facial expression and intonation as information about others' emotional responses. They also develop social understanding and are able to appreciate another person's point of view. Pragmatic awareness of another's understanding and attitude implies a 'theory of mind'. Children with autism or Asperger's Syndrome have impaired pragmatic skills because it is thought that they do not develop an understanding of other people's mental states (see Baron-Cohen 1993).

The main pragmatic comprehension problems arise in understanding underlying meaning. This often involves going beyond the surface or literal interpretation of the spoken words, as in inferring the wrong meaning from another's communication. This difficulty may come from lack of a theory of mind, and is often linked with problems in cognitive, social and semantic understanding (Leinonen and Letts 1997). In the absence of ability to infer meaning, children may make a literal interpretation of language which leads to misunderstandings. Children with learning difficulties or with autism, Asperger's Syndrome and semantic-pragmatic difficulties (SPD) often have difficulties in understanding implied meanings. (For further reading on the SPD debate, see Bishop 1989 and Boucher 1998.)

Checkpoint 3.3

Relevance theory has a possible explanation of why pragmatic behaviours are perceived as a problem in a given context. Leinonen and Kerbel (1999) use this view to analyse where breakdown occurs in conversations and to determine whether the difficulties are related more to explicit, semantic misunderstanding or implied, pragmatic comprehension. They suggest that there is a close connection between cognitive understanding and pragmatic ability. Which of the following two examples are more likely to be a semantic misunderstanding and which is a problem of pragmatic comprehension?

- A boy was having difficulty using irregular past tense verbs appropriately and seemed to be picking them up as we went through various examples. However, he was persisting in using 'eated'. It was pointed out to him that we use 'ate' as the past tense. 'Oh no', he said adamantly. 'Ate is a number.'
- A four-year-old boy with Asperger's Syndrome insisted on greeting me each time we met with the statement, 'My baby's name is Becky.' While this statement was true, by the time I had heard it for two weeks I asked his mother to explain that other greetings such as 'Hello' might be more appropriate to use. The next time we met he had had his talk from his mother, but it had only served to confuse the issue, as he greeted me with, 'I think my baby's name is Becky.'

If the misunderstanding is semantic, then extending a child's vocabulary and using classification and association may strengthen the knowledge of word use and meaning. This area is discussed further below with word-finding difficulties. However, teachers, therapists and parents may need to observe pragmatic comprehension in a structured way to plan intervention, if the problem is with understanding implied pragmatic meaning. *The Pragmatic Profile*, which describes behaviours for different functions of language in a developmental order, is a useful starting point (Dewart and Summers 1995). *Understanding Ambiguity* (Rinaldi 1996) is designed to assess pragmatic comprehension in older children, aged 8–14 years. Using language to problem solve, organise and express thoughts is often problematic for children with learning difficulties, specific language impairment (SLI) or language disorders. Some published programmes offer ideas to structure thinking and expression in activities for developing reasoning (Martin 1990).

Problems in knowing the dance steps

Learning the steps is a normal part of developing pragmatic communication, as well as being a feature in pragmatic difficulties. Some children may be able to manage simple, well-rehearsed steps but problems may be evident in more intricate dances. These include using different grammatical forms and appropriate vocabulary to achieve various language functions. Learning the steps of the dance to *express* meaning may be more easy to help than problems with the music, which is about *understanding* meaning.

The foundations of pragmatic communication develop in the first year of life. The presence of some critical early pragmatic behaviours, such as initiating interaction, 'showing' an object, requesting by reaching and 'sharing', have been found to be good predictors of children's communicative ability at two and three years (Smith 1998). Children who did not use these pragmatic features as often in interaction, showed speech and language difficulties by two to three years. Smith suggests that children influence their interaction environment from an early age, affecting the amount and type of exposure to language they experience in their daily lives. The result is that young children who use pragmatic features effectively will create more opportunities for interaction.

Linguistic behaviours are affected by both language problems and pragmatic difficulties. A general language difficulty which affects semantic and syntactic understanding and use will cause pragmatic problems. Children with learning or linguistic difficulties or specific language impairment (SLI) are more likely to have restricted understanding and use of vocabulary and grammar. For example, children with language difficulties are likely to have problems expressing different functions grammatically. If they know they have communicative difficulties, they may choose to avoid initiating conversations, requesting clarification or giving adequate explanations. Children with pragmatic difficulties often use vocabulary for certain concepts inappropriately. These include space concepts in prepositions, time concepts in sequencing, and more abstract concepts such as metaphors, jokes and idioms. For example, one boy persisted in using 'at the wall' because 'on' could only apply where surfaces were horizontal and could have something put flat on them. Kerbel and Grunwell (1998) cover the comprehension of idioms in an extensive discussion. Some materials are available for use in idiom understanding (Legler 1991).

Word finding problems are also more likely in children with SLI (Hyde-Wright 1993) as well as in those with pragmatic difficulties. Finding the right word is a common problem for all speakers from time to time, but for some children it may have an especially restrictive effect on communicating meaning. The following features are associated with word-finding difficulties:

- substitutions from the same word class so accuracy is affected, for example using 'cupboard' for 'desk';
- circumlocution, or talking around words to self-cue the intended word, for example, 'that animal with the hump';
- overuse of nonspecific words, for example, 'this', 'that', 'thing';
- using gesture and pointing to supplement meanings – moreover, this may not be used effectively by children with pragmatic problems;
- delayed and slow responses, long pauses, excessive use of place holders such as 'Umm';
- 'literal paraphasias' where there are sound confusions (an adult example would be the use of 'septic' instead of 'sceptic'), and 'semantic paraphasias' where the speaker uses an inappropriate word with a meaning similar to the appropriate one (in *Rates of Exchange* (Bradbury 1995), a character describes himself as 'a leading mental' instead of 'a leading intellectual').

Checkpoint 3.4

A 12-year-old girl with pragmatic difficulties said to her mother, 'Remember when I was ill, when I had that fly?' Her mother, knowing her word-finding difficulties, quickly established that it was not a 'fly' and suggested the girl might mean 'flu' but this interpretation was rejected. Eventually as the girl persisted with 'fly' her mother worked out that she meant she had been ill with a 'bug'. Which substitution was an example of literal paraphasia and which was semantic paraphasia?

Word-finding difficulties occur because of poor storage and/or retrieval from long-term memory. Storage problems can be reduced by linking new words to established words and concepts through elaboration training. For example, words can be stored using associations with word classes, or with phonemic cues, depending on which strategy a child finds more helpful. A child who performs well on classification activities may remember the name 'hyena' if she or he is encouraged to think of the category, 'African animals'. A child who is confident with alliteration and rhyme might recall it by associating 'hyena' with its starting sound of 'h'. *Semantic Links* (Bigland and Speake 1992) uses semantic associations to aid word recall in worksheet formats and is also useful to encourage verbal reasoning. Problems with vocabulary retrieval may be addressed by activities in which self-cueing strategies like these are used (McGregor and Leonard 1995). As Dockrell *et al.* (1998) note, word-finding difficulties are more likely to occur in situations with high demands on the listener to process the meaning of language.

Turn taking was discussed above as a skill which coordinates people's contributions to conversation. It does this by integrating prosodic aspects of speech (such its rise and fall), nonverbal elements (such as eye contact) and the linguistic information that the speakers are sharing. Children with difficulties in grammatical or pragmatic understanding will be less successful at predicting when a turn is likely to finish by attending to these signals. They may also have more difficulty in handing over the speaker's role or recognising when it is their turn to speak. Intervention with learning conversational rules is discussed below.

Children with problems in understanding how prosodic features are used to express meaning may fail to use these features to decode meaning beyond the surface content of spoken words. They themselves are also less likely to use these features appropriately. They may show monotonous intonation, inappropriate stress on words, or accented speech, all of which will strike a listener as unusual. There will be nonverbal difficulties too, if eye contact is reduced or if facial expression does not match the language used or the contextual expectations. These features are often a major determinant of how emotional messages are understood by listeners. Thus, children who do not follow the rules may be perceived as inattentive, rude and generally badly-behaved. Initiating conversations may also be difficult for children with pragmatic problems if, for example, they do not use signals such as eye contact to alert their partner to the start of a communicative act.

Problems in partner interaction

Children who have difficulties with the first two pragmatic areas will have problems in partner interaction. Partner interaction may also be problematic for most children with speech and language problems. Interaction is affected, as these children often do not have difficulties in knowing pragmatic rules but may have problems applying them. For example, dysarthric speech and speech affected by hearing impairment are distinctive because they have reduced intonation, stress and other prosodic features which affect communication significantly. Some children who are aware of their difficulties with certain sounds will avoid saying words with these sounds in them where possible, with consequent odd choices of vocabulary.

Children who use augmentative communication often have interaction problems because physical use of a symbol board or technology may focus their attention away from their partner. Eye contact will be more difficult for them, as will picking up feedback from facial expression. Similar problems of feedback exist for children who have visual or hearing impairment. Their partners may need to check back on meaning during interactions. Children with dysfluent speech or a stammer may also have problems in interaction although they have no difficulties in understanding pragmatic rules. Pragmatic difficulties in stammering are discussed further in Chapter Six.

Another difficulty with partner interaction occurs when people do not make good judgements about the amount of information to provide in conversation. Sometimes too much information is given, and the speaker holds the conversational floor too long. Speakers who do this habitually do not have to listen and cope with answering questions. Those who have a general learning difficulty as well as this communicative difficulty sometimes give the impression of being more able than in fact they are. Their eventual response to questions or changes in topic may reveal problems in understanding. There are also people who provide too little information. In that case, their listener is unable to make sense of the communication without a great number of contextual cues and will often need to use questions to unravel the intended message.

A related difficulty in providing information is in making the links between the content of what is said and the topic being discussed. Linking information in sentences is achieved by grammatical cohesion including deixis as mentioned above. Children with SLI have difficulty using these linguistic markers effectively in conversations. Cohesion problems frequently feature in the conversations of children with autism because they may fail to understand that the listener needs this information (Baltaxe and d'Angiola 1996). Information may be irrelevant or tangential, causing problems with topic maintenance – holding on to the thread of the conversation. Typical problems range from not signalling a shift in topic, to returning without appropriate links to an earlier topic which may be understood by the listener as perseverating. As children develop better linguistic and pragmatic understanding, their overt problems with maintaining and changing topic may become more subtle problems of topic drift, where comments are related but are not as accurate as expected (Bishop 1997).

However, judging whether conversational content is appropriate and whether topics are maintained adequately is a complex process (Leinonen and Smith 1994). Inappropriateness in pragmatic behaviours may come from a lack of understanding of the rules of conversation, or a superficial or too-literal understanding of these rules. Bishop and Adams (1989) outlined categories for inappropriacy which can be used to identify topic problems. Children can learn to recognise and use behaviours such as eye contact and turn taking in conversation through activities such as the *Social Use of Language Programme* (Rinaldi 1994). These interaction skills require practice in group situations, where problems of overlap and turn taking are less well defined, and where children with linguistic or pragmatic problems have fewer strategies for coping with interruptions.

Problems on the dance floor

Some children have pragmatic difficulties only in certain social, educational and cultural situations. Vedelar (1996) suggests that it is useful to examine social competence by looking closely at a child's communication skills. This is because language, especially pragmatic ability, is essential in achieving interpersonal goals. Inappropriate or limited communication will restrict social opportunities and in many cases, reduce social acceptability. Warden and Christie (1997) outline curriculum activities to improve social interaction with a strong language base in their programme to teach social behaviour. Smith *et al.* (1997) and Kelly (1996) present ideas for group activities to increase self-esteem and self-awareness and to encourage social language skills. Bilingual children not only have difficulties in vocabulary, but cultural differences may also affect their interaction (Kayser 1995). For example, social differences in addressing adults may make children from some cultures reluctant to speak in class. They may also use inappropriately-formal language forms. The range of difficulties encountered by children with pragmatic problems in schools is discussed further in Chapters Four, Five and Seven.

Conclusions

Pragmatics is about making and finding meaning in communication, and this meaning can be achieved in various ways. Thinking of communication as a dance reminds us that communication is an integrated activity in which the individual parts relate to one another. The components of communication can be compared with the four components of the dance – music, steps, interaction and the dance floor. In dancing and communication, it is difficult to consider the components in isolation from each other. Children with difficulties communicating may find some areas more problematic than others. Unravelling the nature of their understanding and use of purposeful communication is the challenge for education and therapy. By finding out what music they dance to or what steps they know, we can interact with them on a more even dance floor.

CHAPTER FOUR

Two case studies of pragmatic difficulties

Kirsty Gilbert

Introduction

This chapter examines the complex nature of pragmatic difficulties through the cases of two children. Its context is the type of observations and assessments which speech and language therapists (SLTs) use to plan intervention, including educational intervention in schools and specialised services. Each child is considered as an individual with communication challenges which can be understood by informed and extensive observation. The value of collaborative working is increasingly recognised among professionals, but is essential with these children because of the implications of their problems communicating in social and educational settings.

Anne

Anne was 11 years old. Everyone acknowledged that there was something odd about the way she interacted with others, but she was not someone who would automatically be recognised as having a difficulty with communication. However, her difficulties became more evident as she approached adolescence and took part in linguistic and social situations of increasing complexity.

She was referred to the SLT service in the term preceding her transfer from mainstream primary school to secondary school. Her class teacher was increasingly concerned by her social naivety and her poor comprehension of reading. Assessment by the network support teacher confirmed a significant discrepancy between Anne's reading accuracy and her comprehension. Retrospective enquiry revealed that her previous teachers thought she had poor skills in listening and attention from her earliest days in school. Later in her school career, her occasional difficulty in transferring learning from one situation to another was noted. She seemed well-motivated but anxious.

Assessment

Initial SLT assessments

During the first session with Anne, I attempted a formal assessment of language. With hindsight, I would have used a less structured approach. This initial question-answer relationship set the tone for subsequent sessions and made it more difficult to obtain the pragmatic information that interested me.

The Clinical Evaluation of Language Fundamentals, Revised (CELF-R) (Semel *et al.* 1987) was used to assess Anne's receptive and expressive skills. Formal assessment yielded little, with scores on the various subtests clustering at her age level. However, Anne's performance was noticeably poorer on the listening-to-paragraphs subtest. Difficulties with inference and prediction were especially evident. Poor abilities in this area could be linked to the reading-comprehension problems which her class teacher had identified. On the word-associations subtest Anne misinterpreted the instruction, 'Now tell me as many names as you can think of for the kinds of work people do.' She named subjects of the curriculum instead of occupations. Her teacher felt that this narrow interpretation was typical of the errors Anne made in class.

Anne's behaviour at that initial meeting said more about her difficulties than did her test results. I began the meeting with an initial rapport building, some organisation of test materials and an explanation of what would be happening. Then I said, 'We're ready to go now.' At that, Anne left her seat, having taken my statement literally. When conversing, she tried to appear interested in what I was saying, and seemed to realise that eye contact and nodding were important. However, she had not yet worked out that it was important to link them to the context of what was being talked about. This caused a verbal and nonverbal mismatch. During the assessment, she scrutinised my facial expression avidly, looking up after each response made on the test booklet, She was happy to continue only if each response received a positive affirmation. Her over-long and intense eye contact during verbal responses felt uncomfortable. I felt Anne was poor at interpreting nonverbal signals, such as my leaning back in my chair on completion of the CELF-R. She did not seem to realise when the assessment session was coming to a close, by taking cues from remarks such as, 'What do you think you'll be doing when you go back to class?' In subsequent sessions, she showed difficulty identifying the closing phases and body postures that signal the end of topics and conversations.

Anne showed good awareness of social conventions such as holding doors open for adults, but her timing of this was poor. She would stumble into my personal space, and we would collide in the doorway. She found it difficult to walk beside me in the corridor while carrying on a conversation.

Anne was keen to interact, and initiated conversation the moment she entered the room. However, her opening gambit, 'Is that a blue jacket you're wearing?' was a conversation stopper. I was thrown momentarily because she had not taken into account my state of knowledge. I was likely to know my jacket was blue and also to be aware she knew. Also, she had not understood my social role as the adult with responsibility to ask the first questions and establish the ground rules. To rescue the conversation, I confirmed that the jacket was blue. I then attempted to move things on by adding that I was quite fond of it, and by introducing a new topic.

That conversational turn let me glimpse some of the difficulties children with pragmatic problems face. I admire their tenacity and understand their withdrawal. Anne was operating with a poorly-developed interactive script. It was the sort of inappropriate remark we all make when anxious or when meeting someone for the first time. Subsequent sessions showed that this was an initiation she used habitually, varying the colour and item of clothing as required. It made me consider carefully the questions we ask young children and the initiations we make. Anne appeared to understand that a question is useful in starting a conversation but failed to understand that partners also take into account their relative roles in deciding what to say. She seemed stuck with a rigid starter question and had not developed more sophisticated forms. Anne's confusion in receiving mixed messages was also apparent in this interaction. She searched for meaning in facial expression, and my expression had revealed confusion before it was readjusted to verbalise the polite affirming reply.

During the rest of our conversation, Anne demonstrated that her linguistic skills were good. She readily initiated conversation and responded to my questions. However, her replies showed that she did not always take my state of knowledge into account, as she often failed to specify what she was referring to, and to provide enough information. Thus, I had to ask questions and direct the conversation to help me understand what she meant. In addition, she did not appreciate the use of cohesive devices such as pronouns, for referring to something previously mentioned in conversation (see Chapter Three). This made her conversation sound formal and pedantic.

Formal assessment showed that Anne had some difficulty processing longer utterances and selecting relevant themes. She had difficulties in predicting, inferring and understanding causal relationships and reasoning in a sequence of events. However, she could organise and narrate a sequence of events when working with picture-story sequence cards. She followed a simple storyline well, but had difficulty processing lengthy and more complex text. This caused misunderstandings in conversations and making sense of written information. Anne found it difficult to sift through information in question-and-answer tasks in reading if the sequence of the questions did not relate to the order of information in the text. When reading a text or question, she would frequently stop at the foot of the page, as if the page's ending were the end of the sequence of meaning.

Anne often showed lack of flexibility. She seemed mystified if the format of a task changed. For example, she had trouble changing from identifying the odd one out of a set of cards, to saying which items were similar and why. Her responses seemed blocked although she had the knowledge and language to reply appropriately. This behaviour was also evident in class, particularly in maths. The confusion was often compounded as she would not ask for clarification when she did not understand what was required.

Assessments from home and school

Information from Anne, her family and class teacher was an important part of the assessment. Anne's parents were primarily concerned with the difficulties they had identified in comprehension of reading, and the problems with prediction and inference which produced incorrect responses to questions. They were also concerned about her difficulty in understanding mathematical problems. She coped well with computation but did not understand why she was carrying out a computational process in a particular way. Anne was an only child and her parents did not have many opportunities to observe her working with her peers. They themselves felt that there was no difficulty with her understanding or use of language in a social context. They were surprised and rather defensive when I shared my observations with them. Initially, I felt their primary objective in being keen for her to have therapy was to assist the development of her academic skills. Over time, their aims for her broadened, as they became aware of her need for social-interactional skills.

Anne was included as a partner in decisions regarding the input of therapy as she had some insight into her difficulties. She focused first on her reading, stating that she could read well at home and felt that she understood what she read there, but that she had difficulties at school. She knew that others in her class laughed at things, and she did not know what was funny. She was apprehensive about transferring to secondary school because she found it difficult to meet new people and make new friends. As therapy progressed, so did Anne's insight and her willingness to voice her concerns. She became a more active partner in therapy, setting goals and monitoring her own performance. This behaviour increased as she experienced success, as did her self-esteem and her view of herself as an effective communicator.

Her teacher felt that she tried to empathise with others but was clumsy in her attempts. She had difficulty selecting and using the appropriate conversational device. To develop this skill, a situation was created in class where she could be observed working with a partner, in a small group and in a class group. The objective was to assess her verbal and nonverbal language along with her communicative skills in a variety of contexts. The situation was false because I was in class. It was also subjective as I was the principal assessor. However, it was essential to observe her in many different contexts if we were to have a representative profile for planning objectives for therapy.

In a small group, Anne's difficulties with proximity in social relationships were evident. She stood on the fringes of the group, hanging back for most of the time. When asked to participate, she was over eager and would stand too close to others. She did not have an intuitive understanding of conversational distance. Another aspect of her communication, particularly noticeable to her peers, was her difficulty with social use of gaze. The teacher received many requests such as, 'Tell her to stop looking at me', especially from the boys in the group.

During the group discussion, she would reiterate what others had said, and repeat others' questions inappropriately. Some of her comments were irrelevant because she shifted topic and went off at a tangent. Her contributions often lacked accurate timing, which made conversational overlaps frequent. She knew the value of seeking and affirming the opinions of others but did not do this effectively. She was clearly keen to use her communication to sustain and develop her relationships with them but was having difficulty in doing so.

During one activity, Anne made an error in interpreting a word with a double meaning, which caused some laughter among her classmates and confused her. She did not understand the two possible meanings which had resulted in the unintentional joke. Her difficulty in using context and her rigid concept boundaries were evident. She became withdrawn for a time after this incident, and was clearly upset by it.

Intervention

Weekly therapy sessions in school over the summer term followed the assessment period. That initial period set the tone for the interaction, with the SLT in control. Anne remained a passive partner. It was difficult to obtain a balance between linguistic and interactive therapy as Anne required support in both areas, but initially, a linguistic approach was used.

One of the main aims in therapy was to explore the multiple meanings of words in context. For example, the different meanings of 'change' were discussed in the contexts of trains, clothes and money. The use and explanation of metaphors and figures of speech was also incorporated into the sessions. We discussed idioms which Anne was likely to encounter, such as 'to have no time for her', 'to have a go at him' and 'to give her a piece of your mind'. These discussions were themselves fraught with difficulty. For example, the week after learning 'to have a go at him', Anne was confused when encouraged to 'have a go' at an activity in class. Her understanding of the nonliteral meaning had overridden the contextual cues.

At the end of term, therapy continued at a different location during evening sessions. This change of location seemed to be the catalyst for change as the balance of power between us shifted. Linguistic work aimed to develop Anne's ability to make semantic links and to develop her lateral thinking. *Making Sense of Idioms* (Allsop and Woods 1990) and other books in this series were useful texts. Anne was encouraged to recognise and evaluate the relevance of prior information, and go beyond the obvious meaning of words. She became more adept at focusing not just on the grammatical forms of the utterance but also on context and nonverbal cues to help her unravel meaning.

Another aim was to help Anne to continue a topic appropriately. It was difficult to follow the thread of her ideas. She did not always clarify what she was referring to, and at times would go off at a tangent, talking about an apparently unrelated event. This was the case when she was talking about something familiar but not present. She did not appreciate readily what the listener needed to know. Conversational practice was used to help her identify when her listener was having difficulty understanding. Her ability to identify this from facial expression improved. Video-recorded replays of the conversation helped. Gradually, she became more aware of the need to stay on topic. She became better at identifying topic shift and timing her own introduction of a new topic. Less progress was made with identifying and using key ideas in sentences.

Her problem with proximity was addressed as far as possible in one-to-one activities. Giving her direct feedback about how close she was standing helped her to monitor this. Direct input was also given about her behaviour when listening. She tended to apply her understanding of how to be a good listener too rigidly, such as by giving the appropriate amount of eye contact. We worked on how to make clarification requests. Anne was not good at identifying when she had not understood, and recognising that there are times when remaining silent is a good strategy. She had experienced much failure in communication, and so I did not wish to appear negative in giving her feedback. However, she responded positively to comments on her changing behaviour.

A variety of methods was used to help develop Anne's pragmatic skills. The problems pages of teenage magazines were used to encourage her to develop a deeper understanding of situations and of the feelings of others. Carol Gray's (1994a) *Comic Strip Conversations* were used to show cause and effect in conversational skills. Groupwork would have helped Anne focus on developing skills for the social use of language, but this was not available to her. Role play was carried out – an activity which she particularly enjoyed. During role play, she had difficulty knowing what was appropriate to say in different situations, and how to behave in them. Also, in that activity, she identified exuberance as behaviour she engaged in when unsure. Attempts were made to develop her awareness of others' perspectives in a conversation. Anne's own understanding was targeted by taking her back through an interaction, such as role play, to highlight the salient information and the clues available. Videotaping such interventions can be recommended.

Throughout therapy, we recognised that Anne needed more natural communication based on real communicative needs. The class teacher's knowledge of her in a wide variety of situations both in and out of school was invaluable. Continuous dialogue was essential in gaining insight into her difficulties and their implications for herself, her family, her companions and the community.

Outcome

Anne tried hard to be a friend to many in her peer group. Yet she was vulnerable and was identified by her class as such. From time to time, a group of other girls would take her under their wing. She saw these girls as her friends and could not discriminate between them and the class's problem girl who attached herself to Anne, and frequently left her to take the blame for misdemeanours into which she had inveigled Anne.

Anne needed support during the transition to secondary school. She herself felt that therapy had helped her and was reluctant for it to come to an end. She had experienced communicative success which, in turn, had raised her motivation to communicate. There was an improvement in her self-confidence and self-worth. Initially, her teacher had noticed that she frequently made comments in class that produced adverse responses from the others. These reduced over the year and seemed to correspond to an increase in Anne's awareness of herself and of others.

Barry

Barry was five years old when he was referred for assessment at a unit for children with communicative disorders by an educational psychologist and SLT during his first term at primary school. A part-time placement at his mainstream school was maintained, but the majority of his week was spent in the unit. The team there included a teacher, an educational psychologist and myself as SLT. He had been referred to his local health board's assessment centre for autism, but the staff there concluded that his difficulties were not autistic.

Assessment

Initial observations

Barry was a difficult child to warm to. He was uninterested in external motivators. Social rewards had no value for him. 'Aloof' and 'arrogant' were terms adults used readily when they described his verbal and nonverbal behaviour. However, his behaviour became easier to understand and accept over time, as the extent of his communicative disability was uncovered, with its all-pervading influence on his life.

I assessed Barry's language skills using a range of assessments that gave a picture of his development in the areas of meaning, grammar and the sounds of language. He was quite at ease in the structured format of assessment. However, his lack of response to the instruction 'Show me...', when this was used instead of 'Point to...', was an indication of his difficulty with implied meaning. Similarly he made a literal interpretation of an item on the CELF-Preschool (Semel *et al.* 1992). The item was intended to assess comprehension of a negative grammatical structure using the verbal stimulus 'Don't touch'. The child is expected to choose one of three pictures, the correct response being the picture of a boy about to touch a candle. Barry's response was not to touch any of the pictures.

Barry's comprehension of vocabulary was in line with his age. He also used a wide expressive vocabulary for his age. His naming was fast and accurate, indicating no difficulty with word recall. His understanding of syntactic structure was at the expected level for his age and he used sentences which were well-formed grammatically.

His phonological development was at his age level. However his tendency to telescope polysyllabic words was noted. For example, he said 'nana' for 'banana' and 'side' for 'beside'. An investigation of his sensitivity to the sounds of language showed that his skills in phonological awareness were poorly developed. In later schooling, he had great difficulty mastering basic skills of literacy despite considerable help in this area.

Barry had motor-planning difficulties which had a marked effect on his writing and self organisation, and also affected his development of skills in movement and orienting his body in space. Motor ability also seemed to influence his control over his prosody and the nonverbal features of his communication. He had bursts of excessive activity which were in marked contrast to his customary lethargy.

Barry's assessment included observations in a variety of contexts such as the school taxi, visits to the swimming pool, trips to the local park and so on. He was clearly a child with a conversational disability. At a very basic level, he appeared indifferent to people. He was not interested in what others were doing and had no desire to share his own activities. He was poorly-motivated to relate to adults or his peers. He had difficulty understanding the communicative intentions of others, particularly in starting and maintaining conversations. His own communicative functions centred on having his needs met, and he did recognise the value of verbal language in this – the instrumental and regulatory functions mentioned in Chapters Two and Five.

Barry had difficulties attracting and directing attention. For example, he would not use his listener's name: when this was taught as a strategy, he had great difficulty using it appropriately. He was poor at identifying whether his listener was already attending or not, and failed to see why this was important. Establishing eye contact at the start of conversations was taught repeatedly. He adopted this as a rule, but did not understand its value. He also took it to extremes and would force himself into the adult's space, using his hands to direct the adult's face towards him. He found it difficult to identify an appropriate gap in conversations, and to time his initiation of conversations. He did not value the contribution or turns of others. Some of his attention-getting behaviour was particularly intrusive, such as tapping an adult he wished to speak to on the chest repeatedly.

Formal assessments

Joint assessment, observation and discussion were time-consuming processes. The team felt it was essential to agree on which aspects of his interactional skills were appropriate, and which were not. These processes also helped clarify which behaviours should be addressed as matters of priority, and in which order. Additionally, a physiotherapist and occupational therapist were enlisted to address his motor-planning difficulties.

Various checklists and rating scales were used in assessing his communication. *The Pragmatics Protocol* (Prutting and Kirchner 1987) was particularly useful in considering the nonverbal and prosodic aspects of communication. Rinaldi's (1994) *Social Use of Language Programme* (SULP) was used throughout the specialist provision. Barry was rated by teaching and therapy staff on SULP's summary profile. The pragmatic screening form and the pragmatics profile of Dewart and Summers (1995) were useful points of focus for dialogue among teaching staff, therapist and parents. It allowed us to consider different aspects of communication in everyday contexts, and highlighted differing areas of concern. For example, the teaching staff of the service were concerned primarily with improving Barry's capacity to take turns in a conversation and maintain its topic. However, his parents were more concerned about the social inappropriacy of his comments.

Intervention

In the early days of therapy, Barry would rarely engage in direct verbal interaction with another child. He would use an adult to mediate if there was something he wanted from the child. Over time, he became more willing to initiate contact with other children if directed by an adult, but would revert to using the adult to put things right for him if another child upset him at school. However, he became more direct at home in relationships with his sister.

Gradually, Barry demonstrated increasing use of the function of informing, but his comments were often made without securing attention first. In the early days, they appeared irrelevant to the topic under discussion. What he really meant to say was often evident if he was allowed to continue. However, his contribution rarely helped discussion of a topic to develop, or acted as proper interaction among companions. At times, what seemed to be the start of a genuine conversation was just a chance to let him deliver a monologue on his chosen subject of the moment.

Barry made some comments which broke the social code, for example, describing a member of staff as a 'fat old cow'. The surprising thing about this was that he appeared to wish to shock the adult, thus displaying an insight and a motivation that was lacking in other communicative interactions.

Use of the function of knowledge-building (see Chapters Two and Five) increased during Barry's first year in special provision, though his parents felt that he had always shown this in interactions at home. However, his behaviour at home may have been more of a performance than a real information-seeking act. For example, he would ask questions without an apparent interest in the reply, and walk away while the reply was being given or talk over the response. At school, he developed his use of questioning. It was felt that his objective in this was to control the interaction. However, it may also have been in response to the models available. Staff had at this time been considering their own interactional style and had been aware that it was very controlling. Questions were perhaps being used too much as a means of directing Barry's topic of conversation and of clarifying what he was saying.

Barry also became more proficient in his use of the interactional function of communication. He was encouraged to greet others and respond to their greetings. This was a high priority for his mother. Barry's developing skills in this area eased many of the awkward social situations in which she found herself with him.

However, Barry persisted in showing little evidence of imaginative or personal functions of communication. He was poor at labelling his own feelings and those of others. He did not share any experience or emotion unless prompted. His output tended to be factual and he often appeared confused. When questioned about others, he used a repertoire of responses which adults had taught him. He was poor at interpreting others' emotional states. A typical case occurred when a staff member was given a leaving gift. She was crying, yet was clearly pleased with her gift and said so. Barry showed great concern when this situation was discussed later. Crying was associated only with physical hurt in his mind. His own pain threshold was high, and so his perception of the incident must have been especially confused. There were times when he seemed devoid of emotion. He did not express either pleasure or upset. He was a serious child who did not recognise or use humour. Slapstick did not hold any appeal for him and he found no pleasure in verbal humour, such as punning.

Barry needed to be taught to recognise when his turn was being signalled. Work with SULP (Rinaldi 1994) proved effective in this. Later, exaggerated modelling of social interactions was used to cue him in. He was taught to take account of cues within the sentence structure as well as from prosodic features, body language and facial expression.

Barry's own nonverbal communication was affected by his motor-planning difficulties. He had difficulty linking his body expression to an interaction. He found it difficult to give eye contact. He had problems orienting himself towards the speaker. He rarely used descriptive gestures to accompany speech. He understood concrete gestures, such as when an adult touched a chair indicating that he should sit down, but he did not understand more complex signals readily. For example, he did not respond appropriately when an adult speaking on the telephone beckoned him to come into the room and sit on a chair. He had stereotypical patterns of movement, including a tip-toe walk and a facial grimace when self-absorbed.

Outcome

Following intervention in the unit, Barry's response to the communication of others has improved. He reacts more appropriately to the greetings of adults, and has begun to respond occasionally to the greetings of children. However, it is only within a tightly-structured script that he shows an awareness of what is expected in such situations. His difficulties in understanding interaction and language meaning continue to make conversations complicated. Communication is often something which appears easier for him to ignore than to participate in, partly because of his lack of interest, and possibly because it is rarely a positive and comforting feature of social interaction. His progress and remaining difficulties are described under five main areas below.

Listening and conversing

It can be still be difficult to attract Barry's attention. Generally he opts out unless he is particularly interested in a topic. Even when he is attending, his listening behaviour is inefficient. He can give the impression of not listening, but subsequently shows he has been paying attention through his later interchanges in a conversation or activity. He views his behaviour as appropriate because he was in fact listening, and has difficulty understanding that he needs to use listening behaviour for his partner. Initially, he seemed unaware of the social obligation to respond. He would not signal a response when his name was used, even in one-to-one work. He will now direct his attention appropriately when his name is used. He rarely gives a response to a group instruction unless it has a particular relevance to him, for example, at snack time. He continues to have poor awareness of adult nonverbal attention-gaining strategies, and appears confused if these are used. Specific help with how to listen has developed his awareness of what is expected, but there has still been little change in his use of these behaviours.

Barry does not enjoy conversation and makes no attempts to disguise this. He will respond when it has been made clear that he is expected to do so. Yet, in general, he shows little awareness of when communication is expected. He will maintain silences which are uncomfortable for his partner. We now recognise that the adult in this instance will often fill in the conversational space for him, thus doing away with the need for him to respond. Consequently, all the staff now leave the space unfilled and exaggerate the nonverbal features that indicate a response is expected. Activities from SULP, such as modelling conversations, have been used to strengthen the idea of responding to a partner. In school, there was no one person whom Barry liked to talk to as a special companion. If he did want to communicate, he tended to choose the adult in authority. This would also be the person whose initiations he responded to most.

Barry finds it difficult to alter his conversations appropriately for different speakers in different situations. He is aware of status, and will modify his behaviour to some extent when in the presence of an authority figure. For a long time, he ignored younger children totally, and would make little attempt to modify his output of language to their levels of understanding when the staff encouraged him to interact with them.

He dislikes a familiar, motherly conversational style, and withdraws physically if touched in any way. No situation or time seems preferable to him in school for conversation. However, his mother feels he communicates with her more readily during bath and bedtime routines. Possibly, these are times when conversing is slightly less fraught for both of them.

He shows no evidence of valuing the right of other children to have a turn in conversations, or of their contribution to the conversation. He may have been attending to an adult's turn in conversation, albeit with poor listening behaviours. However, he will cross his legs and turn his whole body away from the group when other children take their turn. His posture appears to signal that the other child's contribution is worthless. This response often seems negative and calculated. It hinders social interaction and is proving difficult to alter.

Literal interpretations

Barry finds it difficult to understand what is not stated explicitly in conversation. He interprets speech acts from their form rather than their intent. Thus, he finds it difficult to understand indirect requests even when they are used frequently and when the context is familiar. For example, he has difficulties with 'Would you like to come and work with me?', 'Can you sit down?' or 'We're not finished yet.' He does not understand the implicit instruction but responds literally. This difficulty applies especially to idiomatic language. Thus, he would ask, 'Where?' if his teacher were to say, 'I'll fall out with you.'

Barry is also literal in his interpretation of pictures. Once, he was shown a line drawing of a boy falling off a bicycle. The ground was represented by a single thin line. Barry said that the boy was riding on a piece of string. He has difficulty linking his knowledge of the world with what his senses perceive.

Problems with topics

During the time he has spent in specialised provision, Barry has come to recognise that some contribution is required from him, particularly in one-to-one activities. However, his difficulty with topics is even more apparent now that he does make contributions. He has difficulty selecting and introducing a topic that is appropriate to the situation. He shows a lack of awareness of shared interest. He will want to discuss his own favoured topics and tends to shift conversation towards them. He sometimes vocalises his thoughts in an inappropriate manner, saying things that are hurtful to other adults and children.

Barry displays many problems with maintaining the thread of a conversation, and frequently produces utterances that are off-topic. He often makes wrong assumptions which seem to come from odd associations and reasonings. He produces utterances that do not move the conversation on. He will repeat both himself and his conversational partner for no reason and will elaborate the topic without any apparent conversational direction. He has difficulty determining what information is sufficient, varying between providing too much and too little.

Barry has difficulty dealing with new and old information. As stated previously, he is poor at assessing what his listener actually knows, and as a result fails to establish what he is referring to. In structured language, he can use relative clauses to define his subject, but rarely uses these spontaneously. For example, 'The car is broken' is much less informative than 'The car that I brought to school is broken.' He can also use pronouns correctly. At times, he will give too little information, using a pronoun instead of identifying whom or what he is talking about. On other occasions he overcompensates, as if aware he is required to specify, though unable to apply the rule appropriately. The result is pedantic language which gives him a pompous conversational style.

Barry's output lacks cohesion as he has difficulty structuring his ideas. He will often omit a logical step when narrating a sequence of events. The shared flow is disrupted further when the listener seeks clarification. Barry may not respond, or will continue regardless of the need to clarify. Alternatively, he may contribute after a lengthy pause with information tangential to the original topic. He is unlikely to notice if the listener recaps on the conversation to make the meaning clearer.

Barry has difficulty working out what his listeners need to know, and what they know already. He has difficulty adjusting his message to listeners' needs, and in conveying adequate information. This is particularly evident when responding to requests for clarification. When asked to clarify a statement, Barry pauses and looks bewildered, almost as if he does not know why he had not been understood. He then repeats word for word what he said before. He is poor at identifying what aspects of his utterance had not been understood. He does not monitor facial expressions and body postures for clues to a listener's state of understanding. Consequently, he is poor at judging what has been understood already. He has the words to help explain his meaning, but lacks the insight to do so. He is poor at identifying and repairing misunderstandings. Rarely does he ask for clarification, even when he does not have enough information to carry out tasks.

Understanding nonverbal cues

Barry rarely uses eye contact to signal turns, and finds it difficult to move between the roles of speaker and listener. This happens even when his turn is signalled to him by exaggerated modelling and the use of a question. Generally, he responds when his name is used to cue him in. Now, there are occasions when he has a contribution he wishes to make. On these occasions, he does not wait for the appropriate conversational gap but cuts across another person's turn. However, he has developed some awareness of status and rights of turn in different situations, as he has started to make some attempt to contain himself when an adult in high authority is speaker. He is less likely to violate the teacher's turn than that of the classroom assistant. He is also developing an appreciation of the effect of interrupting the conversation. During SULP activities, he will comment on any inappropriate turn taking by other children.

Barry finds it difficult to identify when a conversation is coming to an end. He does not see the significance of closing phrases. Formerly, he used to walk away before his partner had finished, oblivious to the effect this was having. He will now wait until he is told that it is appropriate to move away – staff cue him in with statements such as, 'You can join your friends now.' However, his body language signals clearly to his partner that he wishes to be on his way. It is difficult to close conversations naturally, as he does not respond to the verbal and nonverbal signals, and is unsure what to do. His turn taking, feeling for the topic of conversations, and unusual prosody make it difficult for listeners to recognise when a topic or conversation is closed.

Barry is also poor at reading the nonverbal language of others. His misinterpretations appear even in response to photographic material, picture books and real-life situations when there are cues to help him. He is likely to discuss a picture with his hand or finger obscuring a salient part. Extremes of emotion do register, but he finds the behaviour of others unpredictable as he does not recognise cues which signal a build-up from milder emotional states. This can trigger high levels of anxiety in him.

Barry has difficulty appreciating how changes in tone or inflection affect meaning when listening to others. He does not recognise an adult's displeasure, humorous teasing or other interpretations of the literal meaning of the words used. His own output lacks variation of pitch, stress and rhythm. His diction is over-precise. He uses intonation to indicate questions and statements, but does not do so readily to signal the end of a conversational turn. Variations in pitch occur when he initiates a conversation. For example, he tends to repeat with rising pitch and volume if his timings are inappropriate and he is ignored. However, he has recently shown more awareness of situations and tries to adapt his output. For example, he will use a whispered voice to make a comment to his teacher during school assembly.

Social interaction

At school, Barry presents as a child whose primary concern is to do what he wants in the way he wants. His interests are no longer as strong and specific as once they were, but he continues to be particularly interested in mechanical objects and insect life. He shows no interest in abstract ideas. Neither is he interested in books, taped stories or picture material. His reading skills have been very slow to develop.

Barry has great difficulty complying with social conventions. His output tends to be neither polite nor appropriate. He does not make use of complex verb forms to produce polite versions of requests, and lacks the insight to see that this matters. As previously noted, he has difficulty inhibiting inappropriate comments. His awareness of self and others remains poor. Improvements are evident in the areas of physical attributes which have been targeted through SULP.

Barry will now play alongside other children but rarely engages in any cooperative interaction. He does not involve other children in his play, and generally does not respond to their initiations. During play, he is usually silent. His play is repetitive, and much of it focuses on violence, such as buildings falling, cars crashing or people fighting. His general lack of imagination is evident from his limited range of self-chosen activities. However, he will now accept adult direction and has recently become more flexible in allowing changes to the rules of games.

Closing thoughts

The case notes of Anne and Barry show that they still have difficult paths to tread in their efforts to communicate effectively. The team who support Anne are pleased that her pragmatic skills have improved, but worry about the future. She is an attractive adolescent who is socially naive. One wonders what will be the interpretations of her over-long gaze in a few years' time unless she learns new styles of interaction. The team who support Barry are pleased that he has learned many styles of interaction in the last year which have helped other people, especially other children, to relate to him more easily. Yet, these styles often have the stilted appearance of learned skills, rather than spontaneous attempts to need and enjoy communication with others. We would like him to want friends, and to have friends. Goals such as these are frequently difficult to accommodate within our current predilection for individualised educational programmes (IEPs). Problems abound in responding to their educational and communicative needs in the rigid rhetoric of the IEP (Goddard 1997; MacKay and McLarty 1999). We need better ways of formulating goals for real life.

More positively, the notes on Anne and Barry certainly illustrate the complexity of pragmatic difficulties in communication, and the implications of these difficulties for life in home, school and community. Yet, they also show how knowledge of communication can illuminate difficulties, and help children to communicate, through its application in observation, formal and informal assessment, team working and reflective teaching and therapy. Therapists and teachers can address the needs of individual children by trying to understand the communication world which each inhabits. We must learn from the children before they can learn from us.

CHAPTER FIVE

Primary-age pupils with pragmatic difficulties

Gilbert MacKay

Opening scene

A colleague who works in a communication centre could not find a book belonging to one of her nine-year-old pupils, and apologised to him. He replied, 'I suppose I'll let you off just this once.' He did not mean to be rude or even amusing. He had imported a turn of phrase he had heard adults use in one set of circumstances into another setting inappropriately. It is not difficult to imagine the effects of such an exchange on someone less tolerant, or someone less knowledgeable of pragmatic difficulties. To use the terminology of Chapter Two, the 'system' that is the communication of the child might have come into conflict with the 'environment' of everyday living, to the discomfort of both.

Introduction

This chapter is built on the experience of teachers and SLTs who work daily with children who have pragmatic difficulties. That experience is presented as a series of short episodes of communication in action. The episodes make specific points about difficulties in pragmatic communication, and about how professionals can respond to them. They are reported in the main section of the chapter, entitled 'Making language work'. Its sequence is based on the seven types of function which Halliday (1975) identified in children's early communication, and which appear in Chapter Two (Table 2.3). For the purposes of this chapter, the functions in Halliday's original list have been amended as follows:

- 'instrumental' becomes 'getting things done';
- 'regulatory' becomes 'control';
- 'interactional' becomes 'relationships';
- 'personal' becomes 'personal identity';
- 'heuristic' becomes 'increasing knowledge';
- 'imaginative' becomes 'imagining';
- 'informative' becomes 'informing'.

Within each function, there are examples of structures which teachers and therapists have created to help children acquire these functions.

An emphasis on functions and structures echoes the systems outlook on communication in Chapter Two. There is no need here for special discussion of the other two aspects of systems – 'processes' and 'system environment' – because there are elements of both of these in the 'functions' and 'structures' described. For example, the case of Iris describes a problem of function – using language to have a need met. Yet, there are elements of process in her new-found capacity to carry messages from her base in the school to teachers in other classrooms. Similarly, there is a strong system-environment component in Jo's café incident. There, the system (of a child's communication) had an effect on one aspect of the environment (the café), and the café made adjustments to accommodate Jo's difficulties with communication. However, Jo's communication also changed following this encounter with the environment.

Functions and structures are useful building blocks for identifying difficulties in communication, and for responding to them appropriately. They also give general guidance that can help professionals make informed decisions about children's educational and communicative needs. The chapter ends with a summary of some of these points of guidance.

Making language work

Communication for getting things done

The purpose of this type of language is to satisfy the needs of the speaker. A simple version in everyday life would be to tell someone, 'I want…' More sophisticated examples include, 'I would like…' or 'Would it be all right if I had…?' These later examples show additional types of awareness, of social conventions and of the feelings of others. People with pragmatic difficulties are well known for the problems they experience in handling such conventions. However, some also have difficulties with the even more fundamental function of making their wants known.

Iris

Iris was enrolled in a communication unit sited in a large primary school. She needed encouragement to interact with people less well-known to her than her fellow pupils and the unit's staff. The staff discovered that providing Iris with a 'prop' to hold would give her the confidence to visit classrooms in other parts of the school, carrying messages from her teacher and SLT. In the early days, the prop was often a letter to the teacher in another classroom. Iris reads well, and so it was possible for her to read the message aloud to the teacher: for example, 'Could two children come to our group, please?' In this way, the action of making a request was enhanced by the use of verbal interaction which, previously, Iris had been reluctant to use.

The letter to the teacher was a verbal prop. Iris has also used nonverbal props, such as an empty videocassette box. Holding this particular 'object of reference' (Park 1995) gave her the self-assurance to approach a teacher in another classroom to ask for a specific videotape. The essential points here are:

- Have a real reason to communicate.
- Use props – verbal and nonverbal.
- Draw on the support of colleagues.
- Show pupils that their communication does influence others.

Charles

Charles had difficulty communicating with others because he was reluctant to move away from one particular place at a classroom table where he appeared to feel secure. He was helped to lose some of his inhibitions about this, under the pretext of taking part in a visual-perception activity. Though not particularly susceptible to group pressure, he would follow the group's lead in a 'transition' activity, moving to sit at a new table in the classroom. In turn, each pupil was given a card with a drawing or pattern, and was asked to sit at a place at the other table where the same pattern had been laid. Later, this task was made more complex linguistically by telling him the characteristics of the images on the cards: for example, 'Sit at the place with four red stars', or 'Sit at the picture of the girl with red curly hair'. The essential points here are:

- Use 'desensitisation' (see p. 67).
- Use peer group influence when children respond to this.
- Coping with small transitions and changes of routine helps to build up confidence for greater changes in the future.
- Use visual information to strengthen verbal understanding.
- Activities for strengthening one function (such as careful listening) can achieve more complex aims, such as reducing anxiety in transitions.

Communication for control

This function is concerned with using language to control others' actions. Words make people do things. Children with pragmatic difficulties experience many difficulties in this area. Some appear to be too shy to go out and act to meet their requirements. Others will do so ineptly. Still others will show poor regulation of their own behaviour. The example of Iris, above, helped her to use communication to regulate the behaviour of another – a teacher in her case. The example here concerns a different aspect of control – self-control. In this case, visual communication is used to enhance control of one's own behaviour.

Gordon

Gordon is typical of many children with pragmatic difficulties in that he learned greatly from the use of visual prompts. These fell into two main groups concerned, first, with the identification of objects and, second, with the passage of time. Attaching cardboard labels to objects and places around the classroom and school strengthened his recognition of words and concepts. However, visual prompts concerning the passage of time made an even greater impact on him. Visual timetables for the day and for the week were particularly effective. Words and pictures arranged in sequence helped to give him a clear idea of what he should be doing now, and what would come next. He needed a sense of knowing what was happening, and that it would come to an end. With reference to the ending of activities, he enjoyed the self-regulation that came from a routine based on the TEACCH approach (Treatment and Education of Autistic and related Communication-handicapped Children). Further details about TEACCH can be found on the website http://www.unc.edu/depts/teacch/. Each activity on his visual timetable was written on a strip of card and attached by Blu-Tack to a large master chart. His task was to remove a strip from the master chart after its activity was complete, and place it in a 'finished' envelope at the foot of the chart.

There is another point in this example. Gordon's pragmatic difficulties with the passage of time concern his development of understanding time and space. Competence in understanding these concepts begins to develop in very early infancy with most people. But here we have a common problem of pragmatic difficulties, showing a delay in the development of time and space concepts which we would not usually expect in a child of school age. To summarise:

- Visual information can be a powerful method of strengthening communication when children have pragmatic difficulties.
- Visual information is useful for strengthening understanding of concepts of sequence, such as the passage of time.
- Communication for control of oneself is as important as communication for regulating the lives of others.

- Use 'search engines' to explore the Internet for other practitioners' guidance and experience.

Gordon, of course, is also learning to use language to control people other than himself. Here is one approach that is used in a number of activities in his school group. Before a child makes a move (such as rolling dice in a board game), he or she has to wait for another child to say, 'Ready, steady, go.' The approach helps to show the speaker and the listener that others' words have power to direct our actions, and that we, in turn, can direct them by our use of words. Words being used to change things are the verbal equivalent of the 'purposeful behaviour' scheme of Piaget that was mentioned in Chapter Two, and which Lorna Wing (1996) identified as being an area of difficulty with a number of people who have autistic behaviour.

Communication for relationships

Do we want people to like us, be wary of us, pay attention to us, or do as we ask? How we say things – our posture, tone of voice and choice of words – can determine the meaning that others take from what we say. It is an area of communication in which people with pragmatic difficulties frequently experience problems.

Andrew

Andrew was unusually shy about speaking to other people. He avoided interactions with them. He became upset and confused if he had to leave his main teaching room. The staff saw the main priority in developing his pragmatic skills as that of building up his confidence so that he would like to interact with others.

He had a fixation on some objects and topics. One of these fixations was on numbers, and that proved to be a powerful resource for building up his self-confidence. He was shown that all the classrooms in the school had unique numbers. With very little encouragement, he was persuaded to lead members of staff and other pupils to particular room numbers on request. Bit by bit, his confidence grew to the extent that he was able to carry written messages to teachers in specific room numbers. Eventually, he was able to read these messages to the teachers when he arrived. Other activities which involved him leaving the room, but with a low level of stress, included bringing back pieces of equipment to the school's open area, that had been fetched from there earlier in the day. Having his name on a label at his place at the dinner table also gave him the extra security that was sufficient to let him sit there without discomfort.

From this episode, the staff learned that pupils' fixations can sometimes be put to useful educational ends. Also, well-planned, short exposures to situations in which pupils experience a mildly-raised level of stress, but through which they know they are supported, can be useful building blocks for exposure to greater degrees of stress in the future. The recommendations are:

- Use desensitisation to combat shyness.
- Use props – verbal and nonverbal.
- Pupils can often understand writing more easily than speech.
- Pupils' fixations can be used positively to help them become more confident.
- Show pupils that their communication does influence others.

Eric

Eric had severe pragmatic problems because of his reluctance to sit in a group, thereby decreasing his opportunities to communicate with others, and their opportunities to communicate with him. He felt more secure in the presence of adults than of other children, and so it was decided that he should sit with two members of staff at his table to work with them. These members of staff were sensitive to his need for them to keep their distance, literally. They recognised that a number of teaching sessions would have to pass before they could sit as close as would be normal in such circumstances, to take part in worktop activities. Gradually another pupil was admitted to the periphery of the group and, again, gradually, the four members of this new group were able to sit more closely together without adding to Eric's stress. Main points would be:

- Use desensitisation to combat avoidance of others' company.
- Find opportunities for small transitions from one group to another, or from one work location to another, to prepare for later transitions of a larger scale.

Ken

Ken could easily become fixated on the topic of football, and would talk about it all day. It was highly ineffective as interactional behaviour for building up relationships. The staff and other pupils reduced it by yawning and saying they were bored by him, when they had heard enough. This underlined that:

- Peer pressure is a useful force for shaping the responses of pupils who respond to it.
- Consistent application of rules by pupils and professionals helps to establish positive behaviour and relationships.

Communication for personal identity

One of the earliest ideas we express is our own existence. Every day, we use language to put our point of view across to other people, and to make them take notice of us. Sometimes we seem to be reminding ourselves that we are here, and that we matter. Our self-concept and self-esteem are asserted. Children with pragmatic difficulties often have problems with their personal identity in a variety of ways. These range from their use of pronouns in language, through to difficulties with body image which show up in forms such as clumsiness.

Ben

The staff felt that Ben had problems with self-concept, not knowing really who he was and what were his boundaries. His level of confidence was raised by ensuring that labels with his name were posted in parts of the classroom and school where his property was held, or where he was expected to take part in a specific activity. Such locations included coat pegs, classroom tables, chairs and his place at the lunch table. This type of activity strengthened his understanding of self and others in general, and particularly of pronouns, which are the grammatical relatives of these difficult concepts.

Ben was one of the younger pupils in a specialised unit. All pupils in his group seemed to be helped by the personal-identity 'Hello' game. The children sit or stand in a circle. All members of the group sing a welcome to each individual pupil and staff member in turn, identifying her or him by name. Each individual has to acknowledge the welcome by saying, 'Thank you' and 'Good morning'. Essential points are:

- Visual information helps to strengthen self-awareness.
- So does drawing pupils' attention to the various settings and locations of which they are a part.
- Exploit games and other group activities to draw attention to the personal identity and characteristics of individual members.

Mike

Mike is one of the many children with pragmatic disorders whose problems with understanding prepositions, such as 'in', 'on', 'under' and so on, overflow into problems with movement. Formerly, he had many problems with clumsiness which included difficulty in positioning himself in relation to others when speaking to them: he would be likely to come too close to them or bump into them during conversations.

His SLT and teachers had good success with gross- and fine-motor activities which they called 'Space Invaders'. In these, Mike and other children would take turns to walk round each other. Anyone who was bumped against in this activity would shout out, 'Space Invaders!', to show that an unwanted contact had been made. In the fine-motor activity, Mike would trace with his finger round the fingers of his SLT or teacher, outspread on a desktop. Again, 'Space Invaders!'

would be called out if he made contact with them. In the gymnasium, various obstacle courses were set out so that Mike and other children would live through the experiences of being 'in', 'on', 'under' and so on. In the process of these activities, the verbal prepositions which corresponded to the actions would be emphasised by the teacher and the rest of the class. The pupils had to try to avoid knocking over barriers accidentally, through paying too much attention to careful movement. It was clear that:

- Awareness of self has physical as well as psychological dimensions.
- Infants learn much of their concept of self from physical activity. This is still a powerful force for learning, even when children are much older and more mobile.

Communication for increasing knowledge

Every day we talk to others, and often to ourselves, to work out explanations and plans. Instances of communication for increasing knowledge overlap with other functions in the notes on several children above, for example, in the case material on Charles, Gordon, Ben and Mike. Here, however, is an example of someone who seems to be going through the motions of trying to add to her store of knowledge but, in fact, is not doing so at all.

Helen

Helen is eight years old and has a pragmatic difficulty that would go unnoticed in a younger child. She asks the same question over and over again until someone answers it, and then will start on a new repetitive question until it too is answered, and so on until adults become impatient with her. Asking questions is good pragmatically if it leads to the questioner's better understanding. However it becomes a pragmatic difficulty when it is a directionless means of maintaining one's place in a conversation, and when this evokes negative reactions from others consistently.

The SLT and teachers working with Helen became quite firm with her, giving clear information such as, 'You don't need to know that, Helen.' In the beginning, this type of instruction ran counter to the professionals' own standards of polite conversation. However, they persevered for three reasons. First, the technique did begin to work when Helen saw that it was being used consistently by all members of staff. Second, she seemed less surprised by this form of verbal interchange than might an adult accustomed to normal rules of courtesy. Third, the professionals made sure that Helen was also told when she showed good use of the social rules of conversation, for example, when they were able to tell her, 'I like the way you are looking at me when I'm talking, Helen.' The main points were:

- The staff team was consistent in its approach.
- Many children with pragmatic difficulties will learn from being told clearly that their communication conforms to rules or breaches them.
- The team learned to use a direct and blunt form of communication, which went against their nature, to ensure that Helen knew when she was questioning inappropriately.
- Appropriate communication was strengthened by letting Helen know when she was communicating well.

Imagination in communication

Children whose pragmatic difficulties are associated with autism and Asperger's Syndrome are often said to have problems with imagination. This complex matter is the subject of other texts which cover it in detail. (See, for example, Howlin *et al.* 1999.) Experience shows that children with pragmatic difficulties can be encouraged to think imaginatively and to grow in confidence as a result of activities designed to make them exercise their imagination. In the example below, encouraging a pupil to think ahead and put herself in someone else's position – and also to put herself in her own position in the future – was a valuable exercise from which she learned a great deal.

Jo

Jo can still have problems of social interaction in public places, but these have improved after a particularly traumatic class visit to a café. The excitement of the occasion seemed to be too much for her. It might have led to a strong reaction from the café staff when they were told by an eight-year-old child, 'Your food's horrible!' Luckily, the waiter in the café had seen this type of pragmatic difficulty in a television programme, and she became a good ally in the unit's later out-of-school activities. However, before these could take place, the unit staff were clear that such visits had to be prepared for carefully.

That process included a variety of activities, with a special emphasis on role play. Jo and others took the part of customer and waiter, were led in discussion about the appropriate behaviour for both of these roles when in a café, and acted out a variety of incidents in which interactions in the café went both according to expectation and contrary to expectation. In addition, Jo (and the rest of the group) were taught specifically in these activities that the behaviour shown on the previous visit was not acceptable. Also, there was discussion about how waiters might feel when customers spoke to them harshly and unjustly.

With this preparation, a later visit to the same café was a marked success. Jo needed a little verbal prompting on when and how to say the right things. She had still not overcome her very fixed ideas about what she would eat and drink on such visits, but coped well when the waiter told her that what she wanted was not available. The unit staff were then able to turn their in-school attention to a different situation, that of helping Jo not to complain loudly when she heard babies crying during a visit to the supermarket! Emergent points:

- Individual work and group work can be used to review unsuccessful interactions, and to prepare for successful ones.
- Careful structuring of teaching sessions can allow pupils to put themselves in others' shoes, even when they have pragmatic difficulties.
- Out-of-school activities are tests of how well skills taught in school have really been learned.
- Interested members of the public can be good allies. However, even traumatic experiences can be used for learning.

Communication for informing

Communication for giving information is one of its most common functions. Sometimes this is for giving people information which they do not have already. Sometimes it is for more sociable functions, as in story telling or maintaining conversations to pass the time of day in the company of another person. The examples below illustrate ways in which children have been encouraged to share information more comfortably.

Olivia

Olivia's pragmatic difficulty is her unwillingness to use speech. Broadly speaking, the tactics of her teachers and therapist are to treat this as a form of shyness which could be worn away by a variety of desensitising techniques. Here are some that work well by encouraging her to take part in giving and receiving information.

At the start of the day, the children take turns to hand out name badges for placement on tables and chairs. The child handing out the badge has to ask another member of the group, 'Is this your badge?' A spoken 'Yes' or 'No', at least, is expected from the child who is being asked the question. 'Yes' and 'no' can be some of the less threatening words to say for people who have difficulty communicating, and they can be used in many different settings throughout the school day. However, it is important for staff not to fall into a couple of traps. First, pupils have been known to 'train' staff to speak to them using only questions which require 'yes' or 'no' answers. Look for more complex responses, even a single-word answer to a choice from two or three options, if 'yes'/'no' has become a pupil's predominant spoken language. Second, it is easy to fall into the habit of asking children questions to which we know the answer already. This type of questioning has a place when helping a child towards the habit of speech, but real power is added to the value of that speech when the adult's question is a request for information which the child alone knows.

Snack time is another activity that has created opportunities for expanding Olivia's range of vocabulary and length of sentences. She enjoys the role of Snack Monitor. This involves her in listening to instructions, which have increased in complexity over the months, concerning the other children's and the staff's wishes for food and drink. She has been encouraged to tell what she has done after distributing snacks, and this has led to her production of increasingly-longer sentences.

Olivia was reluctant to express her feelings, a type of information which is often vital for understanding and building relationships. A useful aid in this has been a face-chart in which the numbers on a clock face have been replaced with facial expressions of emotions (see, for example, Attwood 1998, p. 194). The children point the hand of the clock at the face which best expresses how they feel, and are encouraged to use words to describe the emotion, and also to say why they feel that way today. Parents of some of the children have reported that they now use a similar chart at home to help them understand their children's emotions more effectively. Of course, the faces chosen will force the children into making one from a limited choice of possible expressions but this does not seem to have limited the value of the activity.

The recommendations are:

- Use the influence of the group when pupils are responsive to this.
- Help pupils find a need to communicate – we do not know what they need to say.
- Olivia had a responsibility (Snack Monitor) to communicate. This adds motivation to communicate.
- Let pupils see that their communication has an effect on other people.

Checkpoint 5.1

Draw a larger version of Table 5.1. It contains Halliday's classification of communicative functions. Try to fill in the table with details of a pupil you know well. Which row categories are helpful and which are not? Can you suggest additions, deletions or amendments that make the classification more useful? How well does it compare with Joan Tough's classification (which is outlined in Chapter Two) or with some other system you know well? Should you have a system like this (tailored to your pupils' needs) for your own service?

Communication for...	*Your pupil's use of these acts*
... getting things done	
... control	
... relationships	
... personal identity	
... increasing knowledge	
... imagining	
... informing	

Table 5.1 Grid based on Halliday's classification of communicative functions

Overview – Structures for functions

The case material above included references to a number of approaches for helping children become more functional, more pragmatic communicators. All are familiar skills in the professional repertoire of teachers and SLTs, and this section summarises some of the principal examples.

Desensitisation

This is used to help people recoil less from situations and behaviour which they fear, or which make them feel uncomfortable. Examples appear above in the cases of Andrew, Charles and Eric. The principle is that the child should be encouraged to take a step into a zone that is slightly new and uncomfortable. The power of the discomfort is lessened by:

- the smallness of the step;
- the support of others;
- the undermining of the discomfort through feelings of enjoyment or achievement.

The long-term reward is an increased capacity to tolerate higher levels of stress in the future.

Teachers, therapists and parents use desensitisation all the time, knowingly and unconsciously. Psychologists and behaviour analysts can be consulted for specialist advice on the topic. Ayers *et al.* (1995) is useful for further reading.

Objects of reference

Objects of reference are 'props' that help us to keep focused on an idea or a task that might slip from our attention because of distractions, forgetfulness, apprehension or limited skills. They have been used for many years in work with a wide spectrum of people who have difficulties communicating. They are also used every day by people who have no obvious communicative difficulties, but feel more in control (of situations, others or themselves) by, for example, wearing a tie, a religious symbol, designer labels or a chain of office. There are examples of objects of reference in the notes on Iris and Olivia.

Holloway's *A Rainbow of Words* (1994) gives good examples of objects of reference that have been useful in the classroom. Park (1995) gives a useful academic overview of the topic.

Systematic use of visual information

Visual information in the form of writing, pictures, drawings, objects and photographs can strengthen children's attention to spoken language, and increase their understanding of it. Visual information persists, while the information in speech is gone in a moment. The notes on Charles and Andrew show a simple strengthening of spoken information by visual means. Those on Gordon and Ben show it in settings where it is used to draw attention to important sequences by pictorial timetables – the order of events in the day, and of events in the days of the week. Such approaches can help to bring the structure that gives predictability and assurance when children have difficulty finding meaning in their surroundings.

Further examples of approaches that use visual material appear in Attwood (1998) and Cumine *et al.* (1998). The graphics database, 'Boardmaker' (http://www.mayer-johnson.com/Software/Boardmkr.htm) is a useful resource for generating pictures and icons for home-made visual materials.

Role play

Role play may seem to be a strange choice of approach when pupils' pragmatic difficulties are associated with autistic behaviour. Conventionally, these children have difficulty 'putting themselves in other people's shoes', and that is the type of imagination that is required in role play. However, there is no doubt that Jo and most of the children referred to in this chapter have responded to the approach well, and have come to enjoy it. It is a powerful tool for preparing pupils for social interaction in activities outside the security of the base where most of their formal teaching takes place.

Carol Gray's *The New Social Stories* (1994b) and *Comic Strip Conversations* (1994a) are popular sources of ideas, as are Howlin *et al.* (1999) on 'mind reading' and Rinaldi (e.g., 1994) on the social use of language.

Group work

Many children with pragmatic difficulties have difficulties becoming members of a group, as the example of Eric shows. Yet, life beyond school is often lived in groups – at home, leisure and work. Groupwork in school is an ideal and natural way in which to practise social skills – turn taking, using appropriate eye contact, listening to others, relating to different audiences and so on. The power of the group shows itself in various ways that can help the development of children with pragmatic difficulties.

Main points to note are:

- Being in a group can encourage conformity usefully, giving a child an added incentive to overcome fears and irrational dislikes.
- Children who value the opinion of their group will want to act in ways that please the others.
- The behaviour of the other children can often give good models for individuals with restricting or disturbing ways of reacting in company.
- The group is a powerful medium in which to learn about achievement and about rising to challenges.

Quality Circle Time in the Primary Classroom (Mosley 1996) gives guidance on one simple, non-threatening and effective form of groupwork. Smith *et al.* (1997) are another source of useful ideas.

Consistency

Providing pupils such as Gordon, Ken and Helen with a consistent, predictable setting is important. Some examples were given in 'Visual information', above. There should also be consistency among the service's team of professionals, to ensure that all agree on the aims, approaches and even vocabulary that are most appropriate for a pupil's needs. In such a setting, opportunities arise naturally to strengthen behaviour that helps pupils to learn, act and interact more effectively. Consistency nurtures security which in turn encourages the development of confidence. The confidence to act and interact – to be pragmatic on one's own account – is a powerful force for overcoming pragmatic difficulties.

Attwood (1998), Jordan and Powell (1995) and Powell and Jordan (1997) give advice on a number of strategies for ensuring consistency of approach when children have pragmatic difficulties associated with autism and Asperger's

Syndrome. Leicester City Council and Leicestershire County Council (1998) have produced a short guide that is useful for teachers in mainstream classes.

Daily transitions

Iris and Andrew are typical of children who have been upset and confused by the movements within their classroom, and throughout the areas of the school, which are part of the day for every pupil. Constant change is a fact of life, and so schools must help children prepare for it. Movement from one work area to another may be a small step for an adult, but a large and frightening one for a small child. Transition into larger, more unfamiliar groups may be even worse. To overcome this, one specialised unit, located in a mainstream school, makes sure its pupils take part in as many of the general activities of the school as possible. One of these is attending assemblies in the hall. The unit's pupils attach name labels to their chairs, and carry them to the assembly hall while it still empty to counteract anxiety arising in the transition from their small, intimate classroom to the crowded hall. Later in the day, they have the certainty of knowing exactly where to sit when their group joins the other classes for whole-school assemblies.

Daily transitions are an element in the TEACCH approach. Visit the website – http://www.unc.edu/depts/teacch/ – for more details.

Real-life settings

A number of the episodes in the main section of the chapter go beyond the controlled setting of the special classroom to more open locations in the school (as in the case of Iris) and in the community (as in the case of Jo). Professionals working in a special service should test if the actions and interactions they are trying to teach there, do actually generalise to life in everyday, mainstream settings, and are useful in these. In systems language, this is the test of 'system-environment' interaction. How successful are your pupils as real-life communicators?

Kelly (1996) has good ideas for activities for teaching social communication skills that can transfer to everyday settings.

Checkpoint 5.2

The table below lists the 'structures for support' which were outlined above. How useful have these tactics been with pupils you know? How might be they be used future?

Teaching approach	*Previous use*	*Potential use*
Desensitisation		
Objects of reference		
Visual information		
Role play		
Groupwork		
Consistency		
Daily transitions		
Real-life settings		

Table 5.2 Structures for support

Coda

This chapter has concentrated on two aspects of the systems approach to communication – helping pupils' communicative *functions* to develop by building teaching and curricular *structures* to support them. The other two aspects of systems – processes and real-life impacts – were not necessary components in that context. In practice, several of the examples concerned processes also, because they related to extended interactions. Also, real-life impacts occur in a variety of small to large systems such as a two-person partnership, a family, a school class, the local community and so on. Pupils with pragmatic difficulties live a variety of smaller or larger systems too, over which professionals have greater or lesser control. Our job is to help them achieve as much pragmatic competence as possible in the controlled settings. If successful, these will give them confidence and competence that are transferable to new and larger systems where they will be on their own.

The last message of the chapter is that there is no special magic in the building of successful structures. Through daily practice, teachers and SLTs have learned experientially from their own efforts. They have learned from the efforts of their colleagues also by observing, listening and reading. Skills learned in other arenas of teaching and therapy transfer well to work with pupils who have pragmatic difficulties. In turn, skills developed in work with these children enhance professional practice with other groups. Characteristically, children with pragmatic difficulties lack flexibility of thought and imagination. Their teachers and therapists must have this attribute in abundance.

CHAPTER SIX

It takes two to stammer: interaction factors and stammering

Roberta Lees

Stammering: a pragmatic difficulty?

Stammering, or stuttering,

> is characterised by an abnormally high frequency or duration of stoppages in the forward flow of speech. These stoppages usually take the form of
>
> (a) repetitions of sounds, syllables, or one-syllable words;
>
> (b) prolongations of sounds, or
>
> (c) 'blocks' of air flow or voicing of speech. (Guitar 1998, pp. 10–11).

It may thus seem as if the speaker is unable to initiate or complete an utterance, and sentences may seem very 'disjointed', with much repetition. Stammering usually begins between two and four years; it often runs in families and more frequently affects males than females, suggesting a sex-modified transmission (Yairi *et al.* 1996).

Stammered or 'disfluent' speech often causes a reaction in the listener with the latter feeling uncomfortable or at times impatient and listeners often report a strong desire to finish the words or sentences for the person who stammers. Listeners often show this discomfort by avoiding eye contact, fidgeting or closing the conversation as quickly as possible. They therefore break the normal pragmatic rules of communication. The person who stammers either notices these reactions or, where there is no obvious reaction, 'senses' the discomfort of the listener. However, the stammering individual then lacks the speaking skills to compensate for the pragmatic breakdown caused by the listener's reaction to the disfluency.

The person who stammers will also react to his or her own 'disfluent' speech and it is often assumed that very young children who stammer will be unaware of it and thus unlikely to react to it. Guitar (1998, p. 11) comments that 'Children who are just beginning to stutter may not seem bothered or aware of it, but they often show signs of physical tension and increased speech rate, which suggests they are reacting, at least minimally, to their speech difficulty.' Ambrose and Yairi (1994) investigated the awareness of stammering in preschool stammering and non-stammering children. Using puppets, one which spoke fluently and the other which stammered, the children were asked to identify the puppet which spoke like them. There was some suggestion of awareness of difference in the puppets in these young children, with awareness being more consistently associated with the 'older' children of four years or over. Thus from approximately four years, children are showing some awareness of stammering even if at that stage they have no label for this type of speech.

Many people who stammer report being able to speak fluently when alone or when talking to animals; thus stammering has been described as a 'context sensitive problem' (Rustin 1987, p. 167). The listener in some complex way is obviously having an influence on the fluency levels of the person who stammers. Of course, some listeners do respond no differently to the person who stammers than to a fluent speaker, though the stammering client often expects a negative response. In this chapter, I shall look at stammering children and their interaction with their parents, then with their teachers. I shall also consider adolescents who stammer and their interaction with their peer group and their teachers.

Parents and the child who stammers

As stammering can elicit such negative reactions in listeners, it is understandable that parents often express considerable anxiety if they hear disfluency in their child. Most parents when they hear their child having difficulties in speaking, will want to assist but often don't know how to aid their child to convey his or her message and thus feel helpless and frustrated. It should be pointed out that in young children some disfluency is normal. For example, the young child may say, 'mummy, mummy, mummy, can I go out to play?' This would be regarded as normal, but if the child were to say, 'm-m-m-mummy, c-c-can I go out t-t-to play?', this would be more akin to stammering. A speech and language therapist would carry out a more detailed analysis of the child's speech and using this information along with other factors in the child's background would be able to determine if the child's disfluencies were 'normal' or reflected incipient stammering.

It seems likely that stammering is a multifactorial disorder: some form of genetic predisposition may be present but it does not fully account for the emergence of stammering in some children. One of the current popular theories to account for stammering is the demands-capacities model discussed by Adams (1990) and Starkweather (1990) which takes as its starting point that the demands being placed on the child outweigh the child's ability to respond. The demands usually cited are environmental and self-imposed. These demands impinge on the child's cognitive, emotional and physical ability to respond. Thus, if the parent's interaction style is demanding a level of linguistic competence of which the child is incapable, this may push the child beyond the boundaries of 'normal disfluencies', such as simple word repetition or 'um', 'er' into stammering.

The influence of parental interaction styles in the onset and development of stammering in children has been investigated for over 50 years. Wendell Johnson (1942) proposed his diagnosogenic theory which has had considerable influence on stammering research ever since. In this theory he suggested that parents could cause their child to stammer by reacting negatively to the child's normal disfluencies and indeed by labelling these as 'stammering'. This labelling and parental anxiety accompanying it led the child to try to avoid disfluency and become more stressed about speaking, with the resultant struggle and tension which characterises stammering. This theory, dependent on all parents labelling their child's disfluencies as 'stammering', was heavily criticised and in fact has been disproved. Zebrowski and Conture (1989) found that mothers of stammering children are not more inclined to judge all types of speech disfluencies as stammering. Although there is no evidence that parents in any way cause stammering, Johnson's theory led to a considerable amount of research in the 1950s and 1960s into parental beliefs and attitudes towards stammering. The findings were inconclusive. Following this, researchers turned their attention to the interaction styles of parents of stammering children.

It is not likely that parents interact unusually with their child before the appearance of stammering but the interaction pattern may change after the child has started to stammer. In a prospective longitudinal study in the Netherlands, Kloth *et al.* (1992) investigated the interaction patterns of parents of 93 children. These children when first seen by the investigators at around three years, showed no evidence of stammering. One year later, 26 children were showing definite stammering symptoms. The high percentage of stammering children from this sample was not surprising as the children had been chosen on the basis that all had stammering parents (65 had a stammering father, 23 a stammering mother and 5 had both a stammering mother and a stammering father) and thus were more likely to develop stammering. In this study, no differences were found in the interactions of the parents with the children who developed stammering and those who did not. However, once a child has developed stammering, some changes in the verbal interaction of the child with others may be anticipated. If a child is stammering the rate of exchange of information will be slower and this may cause communicative partners to attempt to increase the speed of the interaction by increasing their own speech rate. Obviously, the severity of the stammer will play a part in determining the extent of change in the interaction style of the child and the parents or carers.

There is no evidence that parental behaviours cause stammering but there is a belief that changing the way parents interact with their stammering child can lead to improved fluency in the child. Bernstein Ratner (1993) gives the analogy of parents having a diabetic child. They did not cause the child to be diabetic but their behaviour, in terms of controlling the child's diet, can either mitigate or aggravate the consequences. Some approaches to the treatment of stammering in children centre on the belief that changes in parental interaction style can lead to improvement in the child's fluency (Rustin *et al.* 1996). This type of approach is based on the fact that a number of clinicians and researchers have tried to delineate factors in parent-child interaction which could aggravate or alleviate the child's disfluency. This approach to studying the effects of parental interaction style on the amount of disfluency of the stammering child may be over-simplistic. This is because it has necessitated breaking down the interaction style into a number of recognisable components which can be studied and changed. However, each aspect of verbal behaviour does not occur in isolation, and one aspect may influence another. One other complicating factor is the fact that the stammering population is not homogeneous. Many attempts have been made to subgroup this population (see Schwartz and Conture 1988). This has the effect that a successful treatment approach for one stammering child may not necessarily be effective for another. Despite these limitations, each aspect of interaction which has been studied in children who stammer will be taken in turn. One aspect of parental interaction with stammering children which has been quite extensively studied is that of speech rate.

Parental speech rate and the stammering child

It is tempting to assume that if one member of a conversational partnership were conveying their message very slowly, then the other member of this partnership might try to compensate and speed up their interaction. In one early study (Meyers and Freeman 1985) it was found that mothers of stammering children spoke significantly faster than mothers of children who do not stammer. Further, when mothers of non-stammering children were asked to speak to stammering children, they increased their speech rate. It was thus assumed that the mothers in this study were attempting to compensate for the perceived slowness of the child in conveying his or her message. Subsequent investigations (Schulze 1991; Yaruss and Conture 1995) have failed to find that mothers of children who stammer speak any faster than mothers of children who do not stammer. However, the difference in speech rate between the mother and the child may be particularly important. Yaruss and Conture (1995) found that the more severe the child's stammer the greater the difference in speech rate between mother and child. There has been relatively little investigation of the speech rate of fathers of children who stammer. In one investigation in this area, Kelly (1994) found no differences in the speech rates of fathers of boys who stammer and fathers of boys who do not stammer. She did note that there was a relationship between severity of stammering and difference in speech rates between father and son, a similar finding to that of Yaruss and Conture (1995). Thus, if parents speak considerably faster than their child, this would not cause stammering but would certainly aggravate it.

One way of reducing the difference in speech rate between parent and child is to ask the parent to slow his or her speech rate. Such modification of parental speech rate has been found to have an ameliorative effect on the fluency of the child. This has been shown experimentally by Stephenson-Opsal and Bernstein Ratner (1988) and by Yaruss and Conture (1995) who found that when mothers decreased their speech rate the children became more fluent. The children did not decrease their speech rate, and thus the difference between them was reduced. Slowing the mother's speech rate may have been influential in promoting fluency in the child, but it is possible that other factors have come into play, as suggested by Nippold and Rudzinski (1995). These might include slower turn taking or simpler language use by the mothers when slowing speech rate. Modifying one aspect of communication often leads to other aspects being changed and thus it is difficult to know which was the most influential factor in promoting the child's fluency. Zebrowski *et al.* (1996) suggest that slowing speech rate influences the child's perception of the parent's affective state. The child may perceive this as a more relaxed atmosphere in which to communicate. To return to the demand-capacities model, it is possible that by reducing speech rate the parents may be reducing the communicative demands on children and thereby assisting them to find an equilibrium with their capacities which would help fluency.

Other aspects of parental interaction and the stammering child

Turn-taking behaviours

Response-time latency

Slowing speech rate may lead to an increase in the response-time latency – the length of time which elapses before the listener responds to the speaker. Bernstein Ratner (1992) found that when mothers were asked to slow their speech rate they automatically increased their response-time latency. This slowing of turn taking gives the young child longer to formulate a linguistic response and simultaneously may create a more relaxed communicative environment.

Interruptions

Interruptions can cause a normally fluent speaker to experience disfluency, and so it has been suggested that interrupting a child who stammers will also exacerbate the stammering symptoms. It is often assumed that 'interruption' means that one speaker interrupts another and then 'takes the floor'. However, 'interruption' may also take the form of two speakers talking simultaneously (simultalk) and this aspect has been investigated by Kelly and Conture (1992). They found that the duration of the simultalk was longer in cases where the child's stammering was more severe. It is uncertain whether this is cause or effect. Teaching children who stammer about turn-taking behaviours is included in a number of therapeutic programmes and will be discussed later.

Parental language use

The type of language used by parents to their children can affect the whole interaction process. For example, if parents use a number of commands and questions the child may feel more threatened than if they use a number of statements reflecting on what the child has said. Again, employing the demands-capacities model, if the parents use complex language forms to the child, the child may not have the linguistic capacity to respond fluently. The type of language used by parents may place the child under some sort of communicative pressure. For example, it has been assumed that asking children questions places them under pressure to respond. Contrary to what might be expected, it has been found (Langlois *et al.* 1986) that children who stammer are more likely to respond verbally to questions than children who do not stammer, who often give nonverbal responses. The authors concluded that stammering children feel some sort of 'communicative pressure' to respond verbally to questions.

No specific type of linguistic structure has been shown to elicit more stammering in the child but it would seem that stammering may be more related to the degree of 'communicative responsibility' the child experiences than to a response to a specific type of linguistic structure. This would relate well to anecdotal evidence obtained from adults who stammer. For example, they are more likely to stammer when they are asked their name. When only one answer is possible the speaker feels more under pressure than if a number of answers is possible. Similarly, he or she is more likely to stammer in response to being asked for his or her address than being asked what he or she thinks of the weather.

Parental nonverbal responses to disfluency

It is often assumed that parents' nonverbal communication styles play a part in at least the maintenance of stammering behaviour, but this whole area still lacks empirical evidence. Anderson in Chapter Three discusses how eye contact is important in coordinating turns and showing interest between conversational partners. She further comments that listeners tend to look at speakers more than speakers look at listeners. This is an area in which it is difficult and time-consuming to obtain objective measures. It has often been assumed that parents or other listeners look away when a child is stammering. However, Lasalle *et al.* (1991) found that eye contact occurred significantly more often during stammering when mothers were speaking to their stammering child than during fluent speech when mothers were speaking to their non-stammering child. The authors suggest that the increased eye contact of the mothers with the stammering children may be because the mothers are looking to monitor what the children are doing when they stammer, or they may be looking to inform the children that they are listening.

Other aspects of nonverbal behaviour such as proximity, facial expression and use of gestures have not been fully investigated in relation to parent-child interaction where the child is stammering. Speech and language therapists (SLTs) often provide anecdotal evidence that parents' facial expressions when their child is stammering reflect anxiety and concern.

Much of the research noted has been involved with the way parents react to the child. The reader could be misled into believing that all stammering children react to their stammering in the same way. Children react to the experience of being unable to convey their message in different ways. For example, some try to 'push the words out', others may avoid speaking and others may cover their mouths to 'hide' the stammer. The way in which the child reacts will also affect how the parents react to the child and thus the process is 'bi-directional'. If the child is young it is often easier to help parents to change their interaction style with the child than vice-versa. Thus, some therapy programmes aim to help parents to change some aspects of their interaction with the child who stammers in an attempt to create an environment conducive to fluency.

Therapy programmes

Rustin *et al.* (1996) describe how the stammering child is assessed at the Michael Palin Centre for Stammering Children in London. The parents are asked to spend a short time playing as naturally as possible with their child using available toys in the clinic room. Approximately 15 minutes of videorecording are obtained but only the middle five minutes are used for analysis. Parental speech rate is assessed and the difference in rate between the parents and the child is noted. Turn-taking behaviours, language use and reactions to the child's stammering are also noted. Considerable attention is given to nonverbal behaviours such as facial expression, touch, gesture, proximity and the general directiveness of the parent. From this analysis, the SLTs select aspects of the interaction style of each parent, which are then targeted in the management of the child's disfluency.

The authors acknowledge that changing one aspect of interaction leads to changes in other aspects and that the whole process is bi-directional. Parents then view the videotape and are encouraged to identify their own targets for change, while at the same time acknowledging the positive aspects of their interactional style with their child. The first therapy session then begins with the setting up of a 'Special Time' task which is a five-minute task in which parents practise making changes in their interaction style with their child, along the lines discussed with the therapist at the assessment session. Parents then practise this three to six times in the following week and write a report on what they did and how they felt about it. This process continues with the aim that the parents will develop good self-monitoring skills. Changes in the child's fluency are recorded over time to ensure that the changes in the parents' interaction style are producing the desired changes in the child's fluency levels. Typical changes which parents might make would be to reduce speech rate and increase response-time latency, and reduce the complexity of their language or the number of questions asked. Alternatively, parents may be given less specific help to change aspects of interaction. For example, they may be asked to be less directive and to follow the child's lead in play, or they may be asked to become more involved in the child's play rather than take an observer role. In these cases, the therapist is attempting to create an environment in which the child feels comfortable and which promotes increased fluency.

Rustin's programme has been described as it is typical of family-interaction therapy for the young child who stammers. However, a number of authors (Gregory and Hill 1984; Meyers 1991; Stewart and Turnbull 1995; Hayhow 1995) incorporate such activities in their treatment approaches. The successful use of family-interaction therapy has been demonstrated by Mathews *et al.* (1997) in a single case study with a four-year-old boy who stammered. His parents were taught to change their interaction styles to create more fluency, and fluency was increased within a six-week period of the parents receiving this information. They also demonstrated some maintenance of this fluency over a five-week stabilisation period. This type of approach is more likely to be effective in cases where the child has not been stammering for a number of years and where the speech pattern would thus not be strongly established. In cases where the child has been stammering for a number of years, changes in the parental interaction pattern could still be beneficial to the child although it is likely that the child would need some additional help from a SLT. To return to the demands-capacities model, it seems likely that.

> For some children, parental behaviour maximises the child's capacities and increases demands only as the child becomes capable of handling them. Other children, however, may have parents whose models and interaction styles are beyond the child's capacities for responding fluently. For still others, parents' models may be highly facilitative, whereas the child's capacities lag far behind the capacities typical of a similar aged child. (Kelly and Conture 1992, p. 1265)

Rustin *et al.* (1996) also discuss how attention is paid to turn-taking behaviours in the home. Exercises may be given to try to establish more appropriate patterns when that is necessary. For example, everyone in the family may sit around a table on which there will be a microphone, real or toy, and only the person holding the microphone is allowed to speak. This ensures turn taking with no interruptions or 'simultalk'. Meyers (1991) also describes how she uses a soft toy called 'Mr Turntaker' to assist the child to understand the abstract concept of turn taking. Only the person holding 'Mr Turntaker' may speak, and verbal reminders are given if a child forgets this 'rule' and interrupts.

The stammering child in school

Some parents report that their child either started to stammer or that the stammer became noticeably worse when the child started school. Some anxiety may ensue and the stammer will become noticeably worse when a child who may already be aware of experiencing some interference in speech, is faced with a new speaking situation. Some children are so aware of their difficulty that they learn to avoid speaking in class, and thus the teacher may believe that the child is very quiet or shy. The child may also have learned to avoid words on which he or she will stammer, although it is unlikely that a young child will have sufficient vocabulary to do this effectively. However, stammering may become apparent when the child is reading or when the child is asked to answer a specific question.

Teachers often respond with anxiety to the realisation that a child in their class stammers. It is then tempting to avoid asking the child to speak in class in an effort to save the child embarrassment. The way in which the teacher responds to the child can influence the amount of stammering the child has in class. Ways in which teachers can work with SLTs to promote more fluency in stammering children are discussed more fully by Lees (1999) but, in general, it is helpful if the teacher can speak more slowly to the stammering child, thereby reducing the difference in speech rate between them. This does not mean that the teacher should speak abnormally slowly so that the child who stammers is made to feel different. The teacher should also try to:

- ensure that the child has an opportunity to speak without being interrupted;
- maintain normal eye contact with the child;
- avoid stiffening body posture or in some other way looking anxious.

If children are very aware of their stammering it is useful if teachers discuss with them the best way to respond to them in class. Children who stammer can often explain that they do wish to be included in class activities, but they may prefer the teacher not to ask questions in a specific order so that they can predict when it will be their turn, as this leads to a build up of anxiety. The British Stammering Association in 1996 produced a helpful videotape on how teachers can help a child who stammers in the classroom. In this tape, there is discussion on a number of interaction factors.

As the child reaches adolescence there are increasing social pressures. Fawcus (1995) points out that effective social interaction is necessary to being part of a peer group. Teenagers spend a considerable amount of time on the telephone, and nowadays this has probably increased with the popularity of mobile phones. Being frequently telephoned is an indication of social status but the telephone is often described as the most difficult speaking situation by those who stammer. Speakers cannot give nonverbal cues to help to convey the message and must rely on speech, thereby increasing the pressure on them. Adults who stammer have often described being unable to initiate an utterance on the telephone, causing the listener to hang up! During adolescence, there are other pressures involving speaking, such as oral exams, interviews for university and learning to speak to the opposite sex.

When speaking to their peer group, adolescents who stammer may not always be met with understanding, and many are teased or bullied. Some adolescents who stammer then withdraw from speaking situations and thus become less skilled in social interaction. This can obviously affect both their educational and their social development. In national English exams pupils are often required to give a talk and one of the criteria used to assess this is fluency. In addition pupils are expected to take part in discussion and how effectively they do this is also assessed.

Weiss *et al.* (cited by Hayhow 1995) attempted to obtain information from teachers on the discourse skills of children who stammer and children who do not stammer for purposes of comparison. They found that twice as many children who did not stammer, as opposed to those who did, were able to make use of a number of discourse features such as 'able to make introductions', 'talk about others as well as self', 'disagree with others'. Thus the presence of stammering and the child's reaction to it can cause pragmatic difficulties which are certainly apparent at adolescence. It then follows that many SLTs elect to treat adolescents who stammer in a group so that they can share their feelings and experiences, and the feeling of isolation is reduced. If stammering begins at around three or four years old then by adolescence the stammer is at least ten years old.

Many treatment programmes do not at this stage target fluency but rather the communication skills of the adolescent. Fawcus (1995) demonstrates poor communication skills to groups of adolescents who stammer – such as, monotonous voice, looking away, taking up a fixed posture – and discusses these with them. She can then argue convincingly that all fluent speakers are not necessarily good communicators and that even someone with a moderately severe stammer can be an effective communicator. Thus, attention to the pragmatic aspects of communication can help someone who stammers to convey a message successfully. Rustin *et al.* (1995) and Stewart and Turnbull (1995) encourage observation and listening skills in their groups of adolescents who stammer. The groups are taught to observe nonverbal behaviour and to acknowledge and reflect on information given. This is all part of the process of improving the pragmatic skills of an age group who have the additional problem of stammering.

Conclusions

Stammering is a communication problem in which the importance of pragmatic skills is highlighted. In the very young child who is probably just beginning to stammer, the interaction style of the parents with the child can help to ameliorate the stammer. Indeed, some therapy programmes such as Rustin's are based on this concept. Helping parents to cope with a child who stammers also gives them the skills, knowledge and confidence to assist their child when he or she experiences difficulties speaking. This is more effective than a child visiting a SLT once or twice a week, with the parents feeling helpless in the presence of their child stammering. It is strongly recommended that children who stammer should be treated as soon as possible after the onset of the problem. Often, family interaction is the preferred approach in this country. As the child becomes older, the pragmatic problems of the child may increase owing to the child's own efforts to avoid speaking or withdraw as much as possible from social contact. Of course, not all children react in the same way to stammering but for those who do, the preferred treatment would often involve targeting the child's communication – pragmatic rather than fluency skills.

The person who stammers and the listener have a complex interaction, but there is no doubt that the listener can affect the amount of stammering produced by the speaker. Some understanding of this relationship can lead to improved fluency for many people who stammer, and increased comfort in communication for their partners who do not.

CHAPTER SEVEN

The school as an integrated support system for pupils with pragmatic difficulties

Libby Roberts

The context

Collaboration and consultation are essential for the appropriate education and pastoral care of pupils with special needs. Collective effort is especially important when they are in an environment to which they have difficulty relating. Students with pragmatic difficulties in communication have problems understanding and adapting to situations around them, situations which may be confusing and constantly changing. Collaboration among family, school staff, and other professionals can offer the pupil support within a stable setting. This helps to ensure consistency of approach, and leads to a consolidation and integration of learning.

Collaborative consultation may be prearranged and formal, but often the most useful information comes from casual approaches. Staffroom conversations are a valuable vehicle for sharing experiences and discussing concerns, and are a force in ensuring that pupils and their families receive the support they require.

This chapter will review the effectiveness of collaborative working that evolved around a project in practitioner research. This project gave the opportunity to address issues that had arisen in a secondary school for pupils with moderate learning difficulties (MLD). Alan was a 15-year-old pupil at the time of the project. His difficulties in effective communication and bizarre and obsessive behaviours had become ever more disruptive during his secondary school years, and had recently been diagnosed as Asperger's Syndrome. The diagnosis was welcomed by Alan's parents, and helped to explain many of his behaviours, but did little to resolve the difficulties these behaviours were causing school and home. The limited information that was initially available to school staff concerning this syndrome, and the pragmatic communicative difficulties associated with it, exacerbated the problem. Teaching staff took a more lenient approach in their responses to Alan when they learned that his awkward behaviour was unintentional and that he could not help acting up. As a consequence, his behaviour deteriorated greatly! The removal of clear boundaries and firm, consistent responses distressed him further. Structure and control gave him a sense of reassurance and security. Their absence made him retreat into obsessional behaviours. Concerns over the effect this was having on his own education and that of his classmates made it an issue of priority, and led to the extended exercise in practitioner research and collaborative working which is reported here.

Collaboration with colleagues: establishing the extent of the problem

Discussion with colleagues, members of the senior management team and Alan's family confirmed that similar disruptive behaviours were being exhibited throughout all areas of his home and school life. Therefore, it seemed important to identify any recurrent patterns of behaviour, and factors influencing them, so that the school staff might assess the implications of existing educational approaches, and the adaptation and implementation of alternative strategies.

All staff working with Alan were interviewed by the writer. This was a lengthy but valuable exercise. It offered opportunities for colleagues to share concerns and relate experiences. It became clear that he displayed certain characteristics routinely, probably as a reaction to anxiety, and that these caused widespread disruption of lessons. The subject areas that appeared to provoke his anxiety centred on activities where he had to show dexterity, control of movement, the ability to work in groups and take part in discussion. Subjects such as PE were especially distressing for a pupil who was clumsy and uncoordinated, and who did not understand the social rules involved in team working. He had excellent reading skills, but problems arose in the English class when he was required to produce creative writing and imaginative work, and to take part in class discussions. The one area where relatively little disruption occurred was in the mathematics class. The orderly structure of the lessons, the methodical nature of the subject and his ability to work independently at his own pace gave him a sense of control. This was reinforced because each exercise had clear and definite beginnings and ends.

After the initial consultation with colleagues, I began an extended period of observation with Alan himself. Observation sheets and pupil shadowing were used to examine behaviour in different contexts, and to determine which areas of school life were most unsettling for him. In addition, I asked non-teaching staff to complete questionnaires and progress charts, as unstructured times were especially disrupted. These approaches to gathering data were again time-consuming; their effectiveness relied on the goodwill and cooperation of staff involved. Permission to observe Alan during class lessons was especially appreciated as it could sometimes be quite intrusive. Indeed, it occasionally added to class disruption. A few pupils were distracted by the presence of an extra teacher sitting at the back of the room. Alan himself often sat back and enjoyed the extra attention he was receiving. Inevitably, some of the observational data were less reliable and valid because of such departures from a normal classroom atmosphere. However, enough information was collated to draw some important conclusions about the teaching approaches used for the majority of pupils with moderate learning difficulties, and how they may cause anxiety to a pupil with pragmatic problems.

Reliance on verbal instructions

Verbal, as opposed to written, instructions reduce additional stress for poor readers, and they constitute the majority in a school for pupils with MLD. Yet, verbal instructions can add to the confusion experienced by pupils with pragmatic difficulties, as they may understand only a fragmented version of what is being said. However, Alan was a highly efficient reader. In his case, the indirect, less personal approach of issuing written instructions appeared to be more effective. He could read them at his own pace, and refer to them whenever he wanted.

Repetition of verbal instruction

Instructions are often repeated for pupils with moderate learning difficulties, to reinforce learning and understanding. Unfortunately, this added to Alan's confusion as he was still trying to decipher and reconstruct the original spoken message. Repetition of messages could lead to feelings of bombardment which, in turn, led Alan to shut out stimuli and retreat into his own world and routines.

Encouragement of eye contact

Sustaining eye contact may indicate that a person is showing attention, and is often taken as a sign of this when teaching pupils who have MLD. However, eye contact was extremely uncomfortable for Alan, and may be so for many people with pragmatic difficulties. As long ago as 1975, Bruner warned against assuming that eye contact had an easily-understood, central role in communication, but his message has rarely been heeded. Alan was able to listen and concentrate better when using peripheral vision to make contact when in company, and reacted evasively to any attempts to maintain direct eye contact.

Use of nonverbal gestures and facial expressions

Some teachers reported that they have found it useful to exaggerate their facial expressions and to use gestures to emphasise points when working with many of their pupils who have moderate learning difficulties. This 'redundant' information (Hsia 1977) helps sustain pupils' attention and interest, and reinforces spoken words. However, Alan frequently had trouble understanding these subtleties of expression, misread the messages and responded in a totally inappropriate way. Indeed, the added stimuli were distracting for him. This note of caution is worth keeping in mind, as professionals working with people who have pragmatic difficulties often advise reinforcing verbal with visual information. Choosing the right visual material for individual children is an art as much as it is a prescription.

Learning by observation

This was another area in which teachers confused Alan by using a technique that was usually successful with the remainder of the class. Often, Alan did not seem to realise that the teacher was demonstrating a task for his benefit, so that he might then follow it through himself. This was further aggravated by his difficulty in transferring skills from one context to the next, such as the context of the demonstration to the context in which he should carry out the task on his own.

Informal approaches to lessons and classroom planning

Group and discussion work involve social skills, such as turn taking, which pupils with pragmatic difficulties are likely to find confusing. They will often appear rude, insensitive and awkward in these situations. Alan much preferred individual tasks where he could work at his own pace without the need to interact with others, and where he could rely on rigid structure for a sense of control and security. In addition, he had difficulty responding confidently in the informal environment which teachers found successful in motivating the majority of pupils. A classroom that is orderly with minimal noise and clutter was not their preferred means of achieving a busy, working environment. They even found that colourful wall displays which brightened up the classroom for the other pupils were over-stimulating for Alan.

Flexibility

Flexibility is essential in accommodating the normal variations from routine that occur in every secondary classroom every day. To allow for school activities such as art projects, swimming galas and athletic events, changes in timetabling are unavoidable. Yet the smallest alteration was seen to cause Alan great distress. He needed the reassurance of being able to anticipate correctly, and rely on a regular sequence of events and routines.

Diffusing confrontations

Teachers frequently rely on the use of humour and distraction to avoid and deter potential confrontations. However, Alan was not easily distracted from an issue that was upsetting him and would relentlessly keep on making a fuss until the matter was resolved. He did not recognise the 'get-out' opportunities that the teacher was offering him by using diversionary tactics, and could become increasingly agitated and distressed.

In secondary schools, pupils travel from one class to the next for each change of subject. In each class, pupils encounter a different set of rules, different teaching approaches and different teacher expectations. More responsibility and initiative is expected of older pupils, and inappropriate behaviours are tolerated less. In these circumstances, it is not surprising that secondary school life can be a confusing experience for pupils with pragmatic difficulties. In an effort to regain a sense of order and control they may retreat into their own world, pursuing obsessional interests and behaviours. These can be easily misinterpreted by teachers, especially if understanding of the condition is limited. Questionnaires completed by teachers in the study revealed that these behaviours were perceived as stubborn, cheeky, rude, time-wasting and attention-seeking – designed to annoy intentionally, and to provoke other class members. Yet, this misconception could not have been further from the truth, which was that Alan was indifferent to the feelings of other people, and seemed unaware that his actions and behaviours might affect them in any way.

Having identified certain areas that aggravated the difficulties already being experienced by Alan, I wished to gauge how effective were teachers' responses and discipline measures.

Addressing the issues

Consultation with assistant head teacher

Discussion with the assistant head teacher (AHT), whose remit included discipline, highlighted concerns regarding the appropriateness and effectiveness of existing procedures. One strategy, most frequently deployed, was to isolate Alan from his classmates, at an area near the main office where he could continue with classwork on his own. This form of 'time out' allowed him to calm down and the teacher to resettle the class. Another consequence of misbehaviour was for Alan to be kept in at intervals and lunchtimes, completing worksheets instead of participating in playground activities. The outcome? Alan found socialising difficult and disliked busy interaction with his peers, and so these punishments were quite enjoyable and often more desirable than the circumstances from which he had been removed. Consequently, inappropriate behaviours were being reinforced rather than weakened.

Another concern was the timing of formal punishment. Often it would be days after the actual misdemeanour. This time gap meant that Alan perceived no connection between punishment and offence. His limited understanding of what constituted 'good' and 'bad' behaviours added to this general disassociation and lack of responsibility for the events surrounding him. In effect, the school's punishment procedures lacked any real meaning for him. He was unlikely to change to more appropriate behaviour because he did not understand what behaviours were inappropriate, or why they were inappropriate.

A recurring slippery slope leading to referral incidents

An important part of my consultation with the AHT involved review of 'referral' data – information on incidents that had caused Alan to be reported to the AHT for misdemeanours. Referral forms are completed by classroom teachers when a disruptive event occurs, warranting further attention. Details of the misdemeanour are described in full. Those relating to Alan were particularly lengthy. Each of his referral forms described a remarkably similar pattern of events.

Most of the incidents began when he was given verbal instructions, which seemed straightforward but evoked no response from him. The teacher would then repeat the instruction, not realising that Alan was still trying to decipher the original message. When there was still no reaction, the teacher repeated it, perhaps with a raised voice or by changing the wording of the instruction, but unaware of the added stress this caused Alan. At this point, he was usually very confused, refusing eye contact, retreating into his own world and shutting out all the disturbing, bombardment of noise. Teachers would interpret this as an intentional ignoring of them, and this interpretation would be reinforced when he resorted to obsessive behaviours in an attempt to regain some modicum of control over the situation. His apparent rudeness and blatant disregard would raise the teacher's level of frustration and anger.

As the teacher became more annoyed, Alan became more agitated, and the other pupils often added to the pressure by encouraging him to follow the instructions. The teacher would then try to negotiate some order with the threat of sending a referral form to the AHT. But this was a verbal threat, and so it was abstract and meaningless. Alan would continue with his 'stubborn' behaviours. As a last resort, the teacher would produce a referral form and begin to write out the details of the incident. The light would now begin to dawn. He recognised the form and connected it with being in trouble, although he was still unaware of what he had done wrong. He would then read the details being written. Because he reads well, he would realise what the teacher wanted him to do in the first place and would begin to carry out the original request. On seeing this, the teacher would think he had understood all along and that he was 'chancing it'. The referral form would then be sent to the AHT. Alan would become increasingly agitated: he could not understand why he was still in trouble, because he had now completed the required task.

Such confrontations between teacher and pupil are time-consuming and disruptive to lessons. Everyone involved becomes frustrated and angry; the other pupils in the class become increasingly annoyed and resentful. Often pupils at the centre of incidents may not know why they are in trouble or what they have done wrong. In the school where the study took place, teachers were tempted to avoid upheaval and stress by referring Alan early in the lesson at the first sign of any awkward behaviour. However, this not only limited the amount of formal education he received, it also did nothing to address the root causes of such behaviours. Indeed, as mentioned above, it may even have reinforced them.

Overall, then, there were large areas of secondary school life which were very difficult for Alan to cope with, and these made him retreat further into unsociable behaviour. All school staff required more insight to make positive educational and social experiences accessible to him, and they required information and appropriate strategies with which to understand and support him.

Consultation with professional agencies

Beyond information from the school staff, consultation with specialist teachers and other professional agencies was required. Speech and language therapists (SLTs) and educational psychologists gave invaluable insight into the problems that pupils with pragmatic difficulties faced daily, and into their distorted perception of the world around them. It became evident just how confusing and stressful school experiences are for these pupils and, indeed, how understandable is their behaviour.

The scope for different teaching approaches was discussed with the specialists, who also offered advice on their adaptation and implementation. Comparisons between long-term and short-term goals were of particular interest with regard to the study, because of the limited time left (two years) before Alan would be eligible to leave school. Priorities included raising awareness for non-teaching staff, class teachers and the senior management team, working alongside each other and with specialist agencies. Information-sharing sessions were suggested, inviting Alan's family and teachers to exchange ideas and concerns. This would also ensure a consistency in the approaches and strategies implemented both at home and in school. Joint assessment-team meetings (of school staff and visiting services) are held regularly in this school, and they allowed all parties to be updated and informed of Alan's progress. All specialists reinforced the consistency with which his class teachers responded to his behaviours. All agreed that this was crucial to his social and educational development.

Collaboration with specialist establishments

Consultations with visiting specialists were invaluable for increasing understanding of Alan's condition, as were suggestions on the management of his behaviour. Opportunities to visit establishments where specialist provision is available were then created to observe these principles being put into practice. Underlying issues such as humour, patience and gentle cajoling all added to the positive and effective working environment that existed. The balance of lesson planning throughout the school day incorporated structure and routine with a flexibility which was included in each pupil's individualised educational programme (IEP). The general approach to teaching and learning was steady, almost leisurely, and this seemed to ensure that pupils were always focused on a task. They were encouraged to work in social groups but also allowed to pursue individual studies. Any niggling behaviour was overlooked by the teacher who used a combination of experience and expertise to determine what actions warranted a reproach. Confrontations were anticipated and, when possible, avoided. Disciplinary reproofs were calm and kept to a minimum, with a clear explanation of what behaviours were unacceptable and why. Cooperative teaching allowed enough adult supervision to monitor any concerning behaviours, and appropriate responses to them, without undue fuss or attention.

Observation revealed how each professional's different role supported and reinforced the work of others, with SLTs working both in the class with the teacher and auxiliaries, and on an advisory level. The visits to well-run specialist establishments helped to show how these strategies could be accommodated within everyday lessons and classroom planning in the writer's school, with minimum upheaval or disruption for other pupils and the staff. In fact, many of the strategies turned out to benefit all members of the class.

Checkpoint 7.1

The subheadings in this section concerned the following aspects of school life:

- consultation with member(s) of school management responsible for guidance and discipline;
- sequences of events that regularly lead to pupils getting into trouble;
- consultation with professional agencies;
- collaboration with specialist establishments.

Draw up a two-column table with these four items in the left-hand column. In the right-hand column, make notes on how these aspects of school life are relevant to any of your pupils who have pragmatic difficulties.

Strategies implemented

Written communications and negotiations

Written communication with Alan opened up unexpected opportunities for conversing with him. The indirect and depersonalised nature of this approach seemed to appeal to him. His ability to read any handwriting meant that communications could be spontaneous as well as prepared. Instructions and negotiations were written on one side of a card. Quite often he would write a reply on the reverse side, reflecting concerns that he had never before expressed. An example of this occurred at the beginning of each PE lesson where, formerly, he would obstruct other pupils by refusing to take part in the warm-up exercise. From his written response to the teacher's instructions, it transpired that he was frightened the other pupils would bump into him as they ran around the gym hall. The teacher suggested that he should lead the run, and from then on he participated fully in the rest of the lesson.

Written instructions allowed Alan to take his time to read and digest their meaning, referring back to the card throughout the lesson when he needed reassurance. Teachers would often refer to him in the third person when writing out these communications and, on reading the card, Alan would score out his name and replace it with the personal pronoun 'I'. This appeared to be his way of accepting ownership of the instruction.

Written negotiations enabled Alan to be taken out on day trips, where previously his behaviour had been too erratic and unpredictable. With exact and detailed explanations of the activities involved, order of events and behaviour that was expected of him, he was equipped with the support and reassurance that he required. The card was kept in his pocket where it could be referred to, either by himself or his teacher, as a reminder of how to behave. Alan would accept even unwelcome information if it was written on a card, although this often involved the card being torn into little pieces meticulously, and put into the bin. We could not be sure if this action was a concrete acceptance of the conditions, or just a show of disapproval. Whatever the reason, it allowed unforeseen changes to be accommodated and prepared for, without a battle of wills ensuing.

Clear step-by-step instructions

By the nature of writing out instructions, ambiguities in them were obvious to the staff, and so they were more inclined to make them clear, precise, firm and in order. This allowed all pupils to know exactly what was expected of them, what they had to do and in what sequence – with a minimum of confusion.

Maintaining consistent rules and boundaries

Alan's need for a sense of security and control was ensured by a clearer knowledge of how far he was allowed to push the boundaries, and what would happen if he exceeded them. Consistency was essential as the relaxing of rules could throw him into a panic. It was not unusual for him to test the boundaries as confirmation that the teacher was still in control. Of course, consistency should not only affect how one pupil is treated, but also how other pupils, and even adults, are expected to behave.

Waiting

This may seem obvious, but Alan required significant time to assimilate information, and further time to form a response and react appropriately. Any pressure or interruption to this process would confuse and distress him.

Time limits

Every task had to be given a time limit. An indication of a beginning, middle and an end helped Alan avoid thinking that the task was never-ending, and reassured him of when he had completed the activity. Even punishments were set within a specified time period.

Positive use of charts and timetables

Charts to monitor progress rather than misbehaviours allowed Alan to be positive about his actions and to assess his own achievements. The recognition of his own progress helped promote more responsibility for his actions and behaviours, and ownership of them.

Detailed explanations

A lack of understanding of consequences, and little differentiation between what constitutes good and bad behaviour means that every aspect of any situation may need to be explained in great detail to a pupil with pragmatic difficulties. Each small part of a process required clarification to complete the whole picture for Alan in this study. The reassurance of when an activity would end, what exactly was expected of him and what he should expect to happen, all heightened his sense of control and security. Although this preparation was time-consuming, in the long run it avoided unnecessary stress for all concerned.

Ensuring understanding

Pupils with pragmatic difficulties may repeat what is said to them, and this can give a false impression that they have understood the instruction. Questions that prompt a differently-constructed answer are a more reliable indication of understanding.

Distraction techniques

This involved the presence of another adult, introducing a totally different focus of attention, so that Alan could be distracted from an obsessional interest. Even then, this proved to be a challenge. Alternative strategies may also be needed as a diversion technique.

Indirect approaches

Depersonalising situations by writing instructions, use of peripheral vision (rather than direct eye contact) and allowing Alan to be focused on one activity while involved in another, were all indirect approaches that enabled him to participate in group work. Also, referring to him in the third person was often an effective means of attracting his attention indirectly. This may seem rude to people with conventional conversational skills, but the repeated use of his name acted as an additional confirmation that the message did concern him.

Use of concrete versus abstract

For this pupil, written words were easier to understand than spoken words. However, spoken words that could be pictured in the mind had more meaning than abstract notions, and were used regularly during conversations. Rhetorical questions, sarcasm and metaphors had to be avoided as these were interpreted literally, adding surreal confusion to Alan's already mixed-up view of reality. Life-skills teaching should involve practical tasks which can be carried out in different contexts, giving pupils with pragmatic difficulties a set of meaningful and transferable attributes. This will help pupils to build upon previous learning, and develop independence for their own education.

Planned ignoring

This can be an effective way of discouraging repetitive demands and constant questioning, provided that no danger is involved either to the pupil or any other member of the class. Although it may appear rude to ignore this attention-seeking behaviour intentionally, we had begun to recognise that it was the act of questioning that reassured Alan and not the receipt of an answer. Often, he would continue repeating the same question, even after the teacher had given him a reply. On these occasions, it was made clear to him that, having answered his question, the matter was closed, and that the teacher would not speak about it again. Any repetition of the question would be ignored. This required a great deal of patience on the part of the teacher and other members of the class, because he had a persistent nature. However, after a few of these encounters, he began to realise that this behaviour was not attracting the attention he sought, and his demands would become less fervent and obsessional. A teacher who forgot this strategy and gave in would find that Alan became more relentless in his pursuit of a response, with his behaviour deteriorating markedly at this apparent lack of teacher control.

Involvement of other class members

Use of behavioural techniques, such as those previously described, required the understanding and support of the other pupils in the class. Their involvement was also crucial in drawing attention to the effect that Alan's behaviour could have on those around him. By heightening peer support, potential bullying may also have been minimised.

Positive use of obsessional interests

Pupils can be directed to use acceptable interests as a positive focus even when they are obsessive, either as a reward for well-completed work or by incorporating them as part of the lesson. These individual interests can be effective incentives to encourage pupil involvement though, of course, undesirable behaviours and inappropriate interests should be regarded as off-limits in school. Alan would accept hard and fast rules as long as they were consistent, firm and applied to everybody in the class.

Keep calm, patient – and persevere

No strategy is foolproof, and not all are effective the first time they are used. It is therefore important that teachers are not easily deterred, and continue to persevere in implementing the strategies worked out in collaboration with colleagues and the specialist professionals. Keeping calm is not only crucial for the teacher's own sanity: any loss of control will be sensed by pupils with pragmatic difficulties. In turn, their anxiety levels will rise, and the situation may escalate out of proportion rapidly. Taking time out to write down any negotiations or instructions will not only give a pupil some breathing space, but can be calming for the teacher too. Having the patience to write out communications and allow the pupil adequate time to respond to instructions, will save much wasted time and frustration in needless confrontations.

Behaviour that can be misinterpreted

Certain behaviours that are characteristic of pupils with pragmatic difficulties have already been referred to as easily misread. Their fluency of speech and repetition of sentences can give an unrealistic picture of what they understand and of how mature they are. Their pedantic speech, literal interpretations, outspokenness and honesty can also come across as cheeky and insolent. The rigidity with which they shut out stressful stimuli when anxious can seem intentionally stubborn and uncooperative, while their avoidance of direct eye contact appears evasive. Repetitive questioning, constant interruptions and persistent demands reinforce the impression that they are deliberately attention-seeking and rude. Misunderstanding rules of how near or far they should stand in relation to others in conversation, and the extent of ownership of a conversation that they are willing to accept or grant, are other social hazards for them. Often they may not realise that they are being spoken to when the teacher addresses the class as a whole, and their failure to respond is seen as an avoidance of work or a delaying tactic.

A pupil's lack of response to encouragement and praise, providing little feedback, can be frustrating for teachers. However, these pupils may be eager to gain peer recognition and may imitate their classmates' behaviour in an attempt to be accepted. Unfortunately, their timing may be inappropriate, and yet again they find themselves in trouble. Verbal disapproval may provoke laughter in the pupil, either as a form of tension release or as an amused reaction to distorted facial expressions. Whatever the cause, this inappropriate response is likely to antagonise teachers further, and so they should be prepared for it.

So, we have seen that there is a range of strategies which are useful when addressing the needs of pupils with pragmatic difficulties. We have also seen that it is easy to misinterpret their behaviours. Thus, it is essential to maintain consistency and understanding in as many areas of their school and home life as possible. For this to be achieved effectively, further collaboration is required by all those involved in supporting educational and social growth.

Checkpoint 7.2

Here is a list of the subheadings of the strategies that were reported in this section. Once again, draw up a two-column table. Refer again to the text, and comment on the extent to which they may be useful for you or your colleagues.

- Written communications and negotiations.
- Clear step-by-step instructions.
- Maintaining consistent rules and boundaries.
- Waiting.
- Time limits.
- Positive use of charts and timetables.
- Detailed explanations.
- Ensuring understanding.
- Distraction techniques.
- Indirect approaches.
- Use of concrete versus abstract.
- Planned ignoring.
- Involvement of other class members.
- Positive use of obsessional interests.
- Keep calm, patient – and persevere.
- Being aware of behaviour that may be misinterpreted.

Collaboration at all levels

Home-school collaboration

The staff found that an open-door policy was important to ensure positive communications between Alan's home and school. Often he seemed to try to keep these two parts of his life separate: home-school diaries proved to be an ideal way of keeping all those involved updated and informed. Two-way communication can allow parents or teachers to work through issues which occurred in another context. Home events might affect Alan's moods and behaviours at school, and it was always beneficial to be pre-warned of any potential awkwardness that might arise in the school day because of these. Sharing experiences and concerns can build up trust, and it is helpful for parents to know that there are others who care. The special knowledge and skills of parents, from their years of working with their child, is essential when devising personal strategies and IEPs. Maintaining consistency in behaviour management can only be effective if continued at school, home and in the community. Without the parents' consent and support, such consistency would not be possible.

The need for support from the senior management team

The consent and support of the senior management team was a critical component in developing whole-school strategies for the support of Alan. Without their appropriate backing and follow-up procedures, implementation of any innovative strategies would have been hindered seriously. Any innovation has implications for the other aspects of the school system, including timetabling and the curriculum itself. There may be a necessity to set up inservice training for school staff. The support of senior management not only provides guidance for them, but also ensures a consistency in implementation and appropriate responses. Approaching a pupil's family and outside agencies can be more direct and immediate when supported by the head teacher.

Collaboration with Alan himself

This may seem an obvious partnership, but it was important for me to remember that the pupil at the centre of this practitioner-research project should not become overshadowed by the process of the research. It would have been wrong if he had been seen simply as an object of concern rather than a participant in reaching a solution. A good rapport and mutual liking is essential between pupils and those offering them support. Instilling trust and honesty makes it easier for pupils to cooperate and participate in strategies, and can encourage them to express personal concerns. Encouraging them to reflect on the repercussions of their own behaviour and their reactions to the behaviour of others, will reinforce the social skills necessary for everyday encounters. Establishing a team relationship that ensures pupils' understanding and involvement in devising suitable strategies will also help teachers to identify meaningful consequences and appropriate rewards.

The use of progress charts and activities based on life skills encourages pupils to take responsibility for their own development, and thereby raise their self-esteem. This may help to minimise feelings of isolation and reinforce social integration. In this study, it proved important to acknowledge every attempt by Alan to initiate conversation, no matter how inappropriate. Praising his efforts often evoked little reaction, but staff learned that this should not deter them from offering encouragement at every opportunity. A strong partnership that fully involves the pupil can ensure maximum effectiveness and success of any strategy, but will require flexibility, tolerance and understanding.

Collaboration with peer group

Tolerance and understanding were also required from Alan's peers, especially his classmates who were regularly affected by lesson disruptions and interruptions. Often the implementation of new strategies worked most effectively when directed to the class as a whole. This not only avoided isolating Alan but involved the other pupils in approaches that were beneficial for the whole class. It also offered opportunities for promoting positive social interactions, reinforcing appropriate behaviours and encouraging team work. By heightening peer empathy and instilling their trust and support, all pupils have a heightened sense of importance and feel more part of the system. This strategy had the effect of lessening any peer resentment of the target pupil when he caused delays to lessons. His desire to be accepted by his classmates had left him vulnerable to being bullied and manipulated. Positive peer regard was enhanced when teachers drew attention to his strengths (such as reading ability), and by fostering an understanding of his difficulties. The support of all class members is especially necessary when new strategies and previously untried approaches are put into practice for the first time.

Collaboration with colleagues

The support of class teachers is required in piloting, monitoring, adapting and evaluating behavioural approaches. This involves time, dedication, goodwill and cooperation. During the period of the study, most teachers welcomed any suggested strategy that might alleviate the disruption in the classroom. An example of this was the English teacher who prepared a card with a list of instructions at the beginning of every lesson. As Alan completed each activity, he would draw a line through that particular instruction, writing any problems he encountered on the reverse of the card.

Having experienced success once, teachers were encouraged to continue using new strategies. Their perseverance was rewarded by significant improvements in pupil cooperation. A forum was established for the sharing of experiences, advice and support, leading to discussion of feedback, concerns and plans for the future. This ensured a consistency of teacher responses and expectations, which is especially important because of the range of subjects taught in a secondary school and the number of staff involved in providing this education.

Checkpoint 7.3

Below is a list of the management issues that were discussed in this section. Draw up another two-column table and comment on the extent to which each of the following issues is relevant in the situation in which you work:

- home-school collaboration;
- the need for support from the senior management team;
- collaboration with the pupil;
- collaboration with peer group;
- collaboration with colleagues.

Reflections on the work-based research

The need for consistent rules and boundaries in all school areas was evident throughout the study. This offered security not only to Alan but also to the other pupils who might have viewed teachers as having double standards because of their focus on an individual.

Some of the simple approaches mentioned in the 'strategies implemented' section proved most successful. However, no strategy was foolproof and certain approaches that had worked previously could become an obsessional focus in themselves. Alan learned ways of manipulating a strategy to achieve a desired result. For example, he might demand a different colour of instruction card, or might score out the wording if he disagreed with the message it conveyed. It was sometimes difficult to remember that these manipulations were part of a quest for certainty and security rather than a malicious or personal provocation. A ready supply of different strategies is useful, and these need constant updating and adaptation.

Implementing new strategies can be time-consuming, but the merits of Alan's inclusion in all areas of school and home life outweighed any initial inconvenience. Changes in routine, although still unsettling for him, could be accommodated if they were anticipated successfully. All school staff needed training in working with pupils with communication disorders, and to have an empathy for their social and educational needs. Alan required continuous education in all aspects of social interaction, and on developing life skills in real situations that could be transferred to different contexts. Flexibility is a key word when working with pupils with pragmatic difficulties, but is not easily balanced with their need for rigid structure and routines.

Any circumstance that threatened Alan's sense of order and control could provoke obsessional and stubborn behaviours, and sometimes escalated into a confrontation between pupil and teacher. It was crucial that the teacher did not back down during such battles of will, or give in to his persistent demands, as his pushing of the boundaries was his way of establishing some sort of security. An understanding of his condition and confusion gave teachers a tolerance and patience with which to form effective responses. Disruptive and demanding behaviours are very frustrating for all involved, but the level of anxiety and stress being experienced by the pupil is likely to exceed any annoyance felt by teachers and other class members.

Achievements for Alan

Socially, Alan became able to relate to his peers, maintaining friendships, sharing jokes and initiating conversations. He took part in team events where he was congratulated for being a good sport. Group work was another achievement, although his participation was often indirect – he seemed to concentrate better when focused on another task. If prepared in advance, he could be amenable to changes, accepting the teacher's decisions more readily, especially if in writing. He was able ask for help, albeit clumsily, and became much less set in his ways, able to release himself from his obsessional interests when necessary.

Showing any empathy for others was previously never apparent but, after the implementation of new strategies, he began to express concern for people's feelings and well-being. The effect of his own behaviour on others still required attention, although understanding of their position was clearly evident at times. He made an effort to show his own feelings, though these attempts were often awkward and clumsy.

A major achievement was sustaining a week of work experience in an office. The environment was both controlled and safe, and his duties were administrative and in line with his special interests. This sense of independence and responsibility was reflected in his participation in numerous community events. Before the study, his involvement in a residential trip would not have been contemplated because of his unpredictable and awkward behaviours. However, with the employment of new intervention strategies by the staff, he was trusted to accompany his peers on a four-day visit where he excelled himself by completing the required tasks and interacting socially at all times.

At the end of the school year, he had achieved Scottish Standard Grade certificates in English and Social and Vocational Studies, as well as numerous passes in modular vocational courses. He has now left school to attend a full-time course at a further education college. The course was devised for students with special educational needs and tailored to allow them the enjoyment of more independence in a safe and secure environment.

Final thoughts on collaboration

Beyond school

The further education college to which Alan transferred already had close liaison with the school in maintaining useful learning for all students. However, for him, the transition from one learning context to another, very different environment, needed to be as smooth and stress-free as possible. Thus, a school representative gave an informal presentation to college tutors to ensure consistency and continuity in appropriate responses to his behaviours. This consultation involved giving information on his condition, its affects, and appropriate techniques which had already proved successful when working with him in school. There was discussion of future concerns, and suggestions were made for supporting him in college. School staff and Alan's parents were concerned that the change in circumstances might trigger off anxieties and cause him to resort to previous behaviours. Preparing him for this transition involved working on skills that would encourage independence and taking control of his own personal development. He visited the college before attending it full-time, to become familiar with the surroundings and his tutors. The school maintained contact with the college after he had embarked on his course, both to ensure a continuity in progression and to reassure parents and former teachers of his educational well-being.

Successful collaborative consultation

Developing and consolidating the structure of support systems within a school relies on the success of continuous collaboration and consultation. This involves creating networks around the needs of pupils, with opportunities for regular communication among their families, teachers and specialist professionals. Reliance on clear objectives with sound procedures and agreed goals will ensure a consistency in approaches and responses. Open and honest discussions that allow mutual support and trust will promote dialogue among all those involved in a pupil's welfare. All parties are kept informed of recent developments, and this sharing of advice, concerns, knowledge and experiences will value the individual knowledge and skills of each participant.

At its most basic, consultation can be informal approaches which develop into more structured team working among teaching staff, other professional agencies, pupil and parents. Beyond, consultation can be a continuous monitoring of a pupil's progress and development, in a search for better strategies and services. This whole-school approach relies on many things:

- the support of the school's management team in accommodating changes to the school's system;

- the cooperation of colleagues who are immediately involved in working with the pupil;
- appropriate training for teaching and non-teaching staff;
- the involvement of the pupil's family;
- effective liaison with specialist agencies and post-school provision.

Collaboration among these will ensure a shared understanding and a consistency in approaches and responses. Every pupil with pragmatic difficulties is an individual with unique needs. It is inevitable that certain strategies for helping them to relate and to communicate effectively will be more successful than others. The pupils themselves may seem to live an isolated life at times, and those who care for them may feel alone too. Perseverance and patience are necessary prerequisites for everyone who tries to support and work with them. Pupils and parents need people who understand and share their concerns, disappointments, frustrations and success – people who know how to listen, and give the added strength that makes them determined to grow.

CHAPTER EIGHT

Systems for establishing and maintaining a service

Jennifer Lundie

Introduction

An effective response to pupils with pragmatic difficulties must be matched by an effective network of support beyond the classroom. This chapter is based on the experience of setting up educational systems for pupils who have pragmatic disorders of communication. It recognises that support for these pupils goes beyond what happens to them in acts of teaching. They need a coordinated framework which involves the classroom, school, their families and the various other agencies who serve them. The chapter will describe some aspects of such a framework, in particular those which have played their part in ensuring that pupils, families and professional services know that they are part of a coordinated team.

Chapters Two and Three made a case for considering communication as a system, and a systems approach to communication appears elsewhere in the book. This final chapter uses the systems approach in a more standard way by examining an educational organisation – the systems that underpin specialist support for pupils with pragmatic difficulties. Reviewing the service regularly in the light of 'systems' questions helps to ensure, first, that it is responsive to the needs of its community and, second, that people understand why it exists and how it performs.

There are many subsystems of a specialised support service that might be considered. Here, we shall concentrate on three which, from the writer's experience, have determined the quality of service for pupils with pragmatic difficulties. These are:

- having a clear *function* for the service. Whom is it meant to help?

- setting up *structures* that will facilitate the smooth running of the service's *processes;*
- issues which determine the impact of the *system* – the service – in the *environment* it is designed to fit.

A clear picture of the service's function

It is critical to define clearly the range of pupils for whom a service has been created. Without that definition, it is not possible to state the aims of the service and, in systems' terms, to know what is its function. Problems of definition are likely to be especially critical when the service has been created by the effective lobbying of a small professional or voluntary group (MacKay *et al.* 1996). If so, a long-term view of the unit's function may not exist. Those who establish a special service for pupils with pragmatic difficulties should have a clear idea of the intended population. If not, a number of issues will cloud its purposes and direction.

For example, pupils with difficulties which arise primarily from their general ability to learn or from their behaviour may sometimes be referred to special services for children who have communicative difficulties. Such a solution may give relief to a mainstream school that is struggling with the challenges presented by a particular pupil. Yet placing them in a service specialising in communication difficulties would be a poor educational decision and a misuse of specialist provision. There is another related danger. Accommodating too broad a range of pupils within a single convenient placement may not allow for sufficient differentiation of teaching styles and other means of support. For example, children with Asperger's Syndrome and children with autism both have pragmatic difficulties in communication. However, the supports needed will not be the same in the case of a nonverbal child with marked learning and autistic difficulties compared with that of an able individual with Asperger's Syndrome. Another example might occur in a language unit, where the pragmatic difficulties of a child with linguistic problems may need different forms of support from those of one who has Asperger's Syndrome and for whom that unit may be a port of convenience.

Of course, an education authority may have decided to respond to pupils with linguistic, phonological, autistic and pragmatic difficulties within one overall service, perhaps even within a general support service. Such generic services may exist for reasons of policy or finance in urban areas. They can be a necessity in rural authorities where the provision of specialised services for very small numbers of pupils is hard to justify. In such cases, it is wise to accept that working with pupils who have pragmatic difficulties requires special skills, experience and knowledge, and that their acquisition has implications for an authority's provision of staffing levels and staff development.

It is important, early in the process of establishing a new service or reviewing an existing one, that clear criteria are laid down for defining its population. Yet, this definition cannot be static. Pupil populations and priorities will change through time, requiring a degree of flexibility in understanding whom the unit may best serve. The diversity of children's needs, communication and behaviour in the population is so varied that too rigid an interpretation of criteria is likely to be counter-productive. The needs of the present will be met by a system which has been flexible enough to be able to adapt to changing demands in the past, and to adapt to them again in the future.

Checkpoint 8.1

If you work in a specialised service where pupils have pragmatics difficulties, consider the following questions with your team:

- How clear are the criteria for admission to the service?
- When is it difficult to judge if a pupil is most appropriately helped by your service, or by remaining totally in the mainstream system, or by having access to some other specialist service?
- What further or additional strategies are used in the decision-making process when appropriateness of placement is in doubt?

If, instead, you work in a mainstream classroom with one or more pupils who have pragmatic difficulties, consider the following questions:

- What specialised provision or support network for helping pupils with pragmatic difficulties exists locally?
- How would you discover if such provision might help you work more effectively with a pupil who has pragmatic difficulties?
- What, if any, barriers may make it difficult for you to have access to this provision and benefit from it, and how might they be overcome?

Admission and transition – structures for process

Context

Pupils with pragmatic difficulties will gain access to specialist provision such as a language or communication unit through a process of consultation and decision making which may have begun months before. That process will continue throughout their contact with the unit. Initially, it may be a means of assessing their response to the service, and assessing its response to their needs. Structured consultation and decision making become especially important during the phase of transition to other educational provision (as a later section of the chapter will show). It may even continue after transition if the service makes outreach provision to mainstream schools. To operate effectively, the service requires structures that will support this process.

Referrals

In the writer's service, referrals come to the admissions panel from community educational psychologists and speech and language therapists (SLTs) exclusively. The unit's existence is known widely throughout the education authority and health care trust. The process is helped when psychologists and SLTs have a good knowledge both of what it may offer children, and of the range of other services in and near the authority's boundaries. Thus, they carry out a preliminary screening of children whose needs the service is or is not likely to meet, before deciding to make a formal referral to the admissions panel.

It is possible to imagine a more open referral system – such as that of the psychological service – where parents, schools, medical practitioners, other health agencies and social workers approach the service directly to enquire about children's possible admission. The creation of such a system does, of course, remove one layer of gate keeping and may, therefore, be considered more democratic. However, such a system would be difficult for a small service to administer and manage.

The composition of the admissions panel has some bearing on the reliability of the decision making process, though there are individual variations in the composition of such a panel. Among personnel included could be a representative of the local authority, a representative from speech and language therapy in the local health board or trust, the head teacher of the school housing the unit, the head of the unit, the educational psychologist and SLT associated with the unit and teaching staff from the unit. Among those invited to present cases for consideration to such a panel might be the child's case psychologist and SLT, staff from the pupil's present school and any other relevant professionals who work with the pupil.

It will be noted that there are two significant omissions from this list – pupils and parents. Both have important parts to play in the process of admission. Rightly or wrongly, experience suggests that primary school children of any age – let alone those with pragmatic difficulties – would be confused in a meeting with a high verbal content and complex social interactions. The role of parents in admissions meetings is less easy to resolve. In the writer's service, parents do not attend the initial placement meeting routinely, though they may do so if this is their wish. However, theirs is the ultimate word on whether or not their child may enrol in the service and, therefore, they have a powerful place in the process.

To assist that process, parents and professionals who may wish to refer pupils to the unit need information. Visits to the unit are essential, though care must be taken to ensure that pupils in the unit are not adversely affected by the presence of unfamiliar adults. Other useful means of giving information include videotapes of the unit, open days and pamphlets.

Part-time or full-time attendance

Part-time attendance may well be desirable for some pupils. It gives them the advantage of access to specialised provision on the one hand. On the other, it allows them to remain part of the life of their own local school with all the social, personal and educational advantages that this may bring. Transition from a specialised service should be less stressful for pupils who have never really left their local school while receiving special provision.

For other pupils, part-time attendance can be a step in the process of transition back to their local schools. Specifying the logistics a phased transition like this might take is an art rather than a science. It should be planned as a collaborative activity at a review meeting in which family, staff of the specialised service, staff from the local school and other professionals involved should decide:

- when part-time placement might begin;
- the period over which it is likely to occur;
- how to balance time spent in school with time in the service over that period;
- how to balance the curriculum during that time;
- how will the transition be supported.

Depending on the service, there may also be pupils for whom part-time attendance in their local school will be an unreasonable aim in the foreseeable future. For example, children whose pragmatic difficulties are part of a more general autistic condition are likely to become upset or uncomfortable when circumstances change frequently. These children may well be unable to adjust to attending two different schools each week. Many autistic pupils require a consistent, highly-structured learning environment. Those pupils are likely to become stressed or confused by attempts to introduce different pupils at different times to that learning environment. Thus placement of such pupils can never be regulated by numbers alone, and all transitions must give due regard to all pupils and be part of a planned programme of support and intervention.

Collaboration and transition

In recent years, policies for inclusion have prevailed in local and central government. In principle, all pupils attending a school should be included in all its main routines. Achieving this for pupils with pragmatic difficulties is a goal whose possibility may be tested readily when specialist provision is located in a mainstream school.

Access to classes in the mainstream of the school depends on the needs of the individual pupil. Consideration has to be given to whether the pupil should be included as an individual or as part of a group. Factors which need to be taken into account include age group (which may or may not be the same as that of the pupil in question), interest level, subject area, social group and so on. It should be a gradual process. 'Readiness' should be defined, and discussion should centre on unit pupils, mainstream pupils, staff and parents. There are obvious implications for staff development. Unit staff should think carefully about the criteria which define readiness. The process must be structured. It may need to begin within the unit, for example, by inviting mainstream pupils to take part in planned activities in the 'home ground' of the unit pupil. It may be necessary to work quite gradually from this starting point towards the unit pupil working in the mainstream class with the mainstream teacher. It will be necessary to maintain a high level of support until the pupil is comfortable enough for this to decrease (again gradually). Only when the pupil is able to be a confident participant in the new setting without support should other areas for inclusion be considered.

A similar process to that described above is followed when children are ready to re-enter or spend more time in their local mainstream school. This process is more complicated and difficult than transition from the classrooms of a unit to the classrooms of its host school. Close collaboration is essential for all staff to prepare (if necessary, by undertaking inservice), to observe, to liaise and to plan. Additional staffing deployed on an 'outreach' basis can form a part of the solution.

Discharge

Any service should have clear expectations about what it is expected to provide and what will happen next. It may be that pupils will remain within the service and that there will be a linked next step, such as a move from a specialist primary into a specialist secondary provision. However, the reality may be less straightforward. Pupils may move into the school which hosts the unit, or they may move into a different school. Whatever the change, all aspects need to be clearly defined and structured.

Building systems for pupils with pragmatic difficulties

Valuing existing professionals

One of the most valuable assets to emerge in setting up a service is the experience gained by those involved in it, simply by working there. This lets them build up a craft knowledge of responses to the communicative, educational and social needs of pupils. It also provides a resource for policy makers because of their unique understanding of:

- whom the unit is likely to help most effectively;
- the merits of full-time placement or part-time placement for different individuals;
- whom the unit may not be able to help;
- how to develop an appropriate curriculum;
- how it may extend its service;
- how the unit's staff, pupils and parents should relate to the staff, pupils and parents of the mainstream school in which it is based;
- how local schools influence the unit, and are influenced by it.

Their experience with pupils who have such difficulties in communication is a real resource. Consultation with day-to-day practitioners should be an essential part of building practice and policy.

Working with parents

It is now something of a cliché to say that the relationships between parents and a specialised service must be a partnership, but it is true nonetheless. Each depends on information and support from the other. Workable systems for communication are essential, so that parents know what is happening at school and schools know what is happening at home. If an information system is successful, both parties will feel supported. Parents are involved in the education of their child and should have confidence in the quality of that education and in the value placed on their knowledge.

Formal methods such as review meetings have a place in exchanging information between service and home, but it is often the case that more informal types of communication offer the greatest scope. For instance:

- Telephone links are essential. It is difficult to commit some thoughts to paper, particularly those which are sensitive or have the potential to be misconstrued, because the pragmatics of writing are different from the pragmatics of conversation.

- Home visits can be important. Many parents and professionals find that the less formal surroundings of home provide a valuable setting for reviewing and planning the support of pupils.
- Other parents find that acting as a parent helper in school is a useful learning experience. However, it may be advisable to have a policy on whether or not parents should work with their own children in such arrangements.
- Parent groups often provide invaluable support, when only another parent can have the necessary insight, through experience, into particular needs and circumstances.

A relevant curriculum

The curriculum aims to prepare pupils for life. Therefore it should be relevant to life at home, in school and in the outside world. It will be possible to promote progress with many pupils by working on specific areas of language or communication. The curriculum will have to be individualised for each pupil within the unit. Its content should be determined by the multidisciplinary team (made up of parents and all staff working with the pupil). It should be based on a thorough assessment of the pupils using a variety of methods, including observation, carried out by those who know them best. Priorities for working need to be identified and strategies discussed.

Yet the nature of pragmatic difficulties demands a degree of flexibility. The special interest or motivator of the pupil could suddenly change, or a sudden surge of learning in a particular area could make a proposed timescale inappropriate for existing plans and targets. Whatever the content, the curriculum will extend beyond the normal boundaries of school into the home and community. There may be subtle changes in the balance of the curriculum as the pupil progresses. It is often difficult to tailor this to individual specifications because of current curriculum prescriptives on time allocations for specific subject areas. However, it is possible to use communication or personal and social education – key areas when pupils have pragmatic difficulties – as a vehicle through which the other aspects of the curriculum can have their required proportions.

Self evaluation

There has been external evaluation of UK educational services since their creation over a hundred years ago. But there is a need for self evaluation too, with all professionals in the multidisciplinary team taking part in routine reviews of their own service. This is to ensure that aims are being met, and that practices and policies may be developed to take account of changing circumstances, insights and the population served. There will be a variety of methods, both formal and informal through which data can be gathered. These include notes from formal review meetings, telephone conversations, home-school diaries, home visits and support groups.

Another useful source of evaluation data is the individualised educational programme (IEP). This import from American legislation of the 1970s has found a place in the United Kingdom, particularly within the last decade (Goddard 1997). The essential purpose of the IEP is to bring control and direction to the education of pupils with special needs, by planning responses to these needs over a relatively short timescale such as three months or a school term. In addition, British IEPs are expected to show how children's targets are in line with national curricular imperatives, namely the National Curriculum in England and Wales, the 5–14 Curriculum in Scotland and the Northern Ireland Curriculum. It would be fair to say that the quality and success of IEPs and similar exercises in goal setting is an indicator of the competence of the goal setters. As such, IEP records are themselves important evidence for the evaluation of the service.

Some of the most valid assessments of quality of service are likely to be made in circumstances where no formal procedures have been set up. These indicators appear in, for example, the comments of parents, families, the pupils themselves, visiting professionals and members of the public. Attention will be drawn to aspects of life in the service which indicate that it is meeting its aims in the setting of real life.

Data from sources suggested in the paragraphs above should be reflected on routinely over the course of the school year. This will help the service's team to gauge:

- how well they are responding to the needs of pupils and their families;
- how they may be judged in the current educational climate and its requirements for easily-measured achievement;
- how the service might respond to the above needs more effectively, and to developments in knowledge of the professional field.

Priorities for development of services

This chapter has focused on the needs of a unit located in a primary school, but it is worth drawing attention to some other areas in which there may be a need for specialised provision for children with pragmatic difficulties. These areas include: preschool education, secondary education and outreach to other mainstream schools.

Many parts of the UK now have an extensive range of services in the health and education sectors where professionals are able to identify preschool children with severe difficulties in communication. The existence of units in primary schools raises questions about the place of the current generic preschool services in responding to these children's needs. Certainly, speech and language therapy is widely available but that, on its own, is of a different nature from the interdisciplinary, whole-day provision that units make for children of school age. However, should children with severe communicative difficulties have to wait for school entry before they have daily help from a specialised service? This is not an easy question to answer.

There can be an equally difficult problem to address at the end of primary school, if there is no comparable service for pupils when they are of secondary school age. Many pupils may grow in confidence and communicative confidence to such an extent that their future education will take place, with or without special support, in a mainstream secondary school. Yet, there will undoubtedly be a number of pupils whose pragmatic difficulties will persist to such an extent that recognition of these difficulties, and provision for them, will be necessary if they are to secure their right to education.

The issue of part-time placement and full-time placement has been raised earlier, and is related to the issue of defining a unit's population carefully. Pupils with pragmatic difficulties are not a narrowly defined group in terms of how their difficulties affect their ability to communicate. Their needs vary, as do the teaching approaches best suited to address them. Some may require a different type of specialism from that which the unit offers. Others have educational and social needs which will always be met best in a mainstream school. In some cases, these pupils will be served well by their class teachers or by a generic learning-support service. Some, however, will need, and their teachers and families will need, assistance in mainstream school that draws on the experience of the unit's staff. Sharing this experience with mainstream teachers is a core element of transition from unit to school. Engaging in that process has shown mainstream and unit staff that specialised experience is a resource which, through outreach collaboration, can be put to the use of pupils who have no need for even part-time attendance at a unit. Exploring the feasibility of such a development is a priority for ensuring the quality of such a unit's service to its community.

Looking ahead

Units for pupils with difficulties in communication are still relatively few in number. Staff in such services should be aware of the problems of working in isolation. They should open and maintain links with similar establishments for networking and staff development. In addition, knowledge and understanding of what is happening in other services lets them have a broader picture of their own field. Thus, they can take better decisions about how to work with their pupils, collaborate with other professionals and devise more effective ways of interpreting the curriculum.

Looking outward strengthens the most important resource of a service – the community which comprises the staff, the pupils and their families. That is the structure in which processes grow to let the functions, or aims, of the service be achieved. It is built on the trust and confidence which come from responding to challenges that have arisen in the relationship. Ultimately, it will determine how good is the service in its interaction with the environment of the wider world to which the pupils need access.

Checkpoint 8.2

This chart refers to subsection headings in this chapter. It may be a useful staff development or individual exercise to apply them to the circumstances in which you work. Draw up a larger version of Table 8.2. To what extent are the issues relevant to your circumstances and needs? Record any priorities in the left-hand blank column. Then note in the middle column any barriers which make it difficult to address these priorities as satisfactorily as you wish. Finally, make proposals for overcoming the barriers.

Issue	*Priorities*	*Barriers*	*Solutions*
Referrals			
Part-time or full-time attendance			
Collaboration and transition			
Discharge			
Valuing existing professionals			
Working with parents			
A relevant curriculum			
Evaluation			

Table 8.2 Chart for staff development exercise

References

Adams, M. (1990) 'The demands and capacities model I: theoretical elaborations', *Journal of Fluency Disorders* **15**(2), 135–41.

Allsop, J. and Woods, L. (1990) *Making Sense of Idioms*. London: Cassell.

Ambrose, N. G. and Yairi, E. (1994) 'The development of awareness of stuttering in preschool children', *Journal of Fluency Disorders* **19**(2), 229–45.

Arkell, J. E. H. (1986) 'The language teaching device', *Child: Care, Health and Development* **12**(3), 151–66.

Attwood, T. (1998) *Asperger's Syndrome*. London: Jessica Kingsley.

Austin, J. L. (1962) *How to do Things with Words*. Oxford: Oxford University Press.

Ayers, H. *et al.* (1995) *Perspectives on Behaviour: A Practical Guide to Effective Intervention for Teachers*. London: David Fulton Publishers.

Bachman, L. F. (1990) *Fundamental Considerations in Language Testing*. Oxford: Oxford University Press.

Baltaxe, C. and d'Angiola, N. (1996) 'Referencing skills in children with autism and specific language impairment', *European Journal of Disorders of Communication* **31**(3), 245–58.

Banathy, B. H. (1973) *Developing a Systems View of Education: The Systems Model Approach*. Belmont, CA: Lear Siegler Inc.

Banathy, B. H. (1992) *A Systems View of Education: Concepts and Principles for Effective Practice*. Englewood Cliffs, NJ: Educational Technology Publications.

Banathy, B. H. (1996) *Designing Social Systems in a Changing World*. New York: Plenum Press.

Baron-Cohen, S. (1993) *Understanding Others' Minds*. Oxford: Oxford University Press.

Bates, E. and MacWhinney, B. (1979) 'A functionalist approach to the acquisition of grammar', in Ochs, E. and Schiefflin, B. (eds) *Developmental Pragmatics*, 167–211. New York: Academic Press.

Bernstein Ratner, N. (1992) 'Measurable outcomes of instructions to modify normal parent-child verbal interactions: Implications for indirect stuttering therapy', *Journal of Speech and Hearing Research* **35**(1), 14–20.

Bernstein Ratner, N. (1993) 'Parents, children and stuttering', *Seminars in Speech and Language* **14**(3), 238–49.

Bigland, S. and Speake, J. (1992) *Semantic Links.* Bicester, Oxford: Winslow.

Bishop, D. V. M. (1989) 'Autism, Asperger's Syndrome and semantic pragmatic disorder: where are the boundaries?' *British Journal of Disorders of Communication* **24**(2), 107–21.

Bishop, D. V. M. (1997) *Uncommon Understanding.* Hove: Psychology Press.

Bishop, D. V. M. and Adams, C. (1989) 'Conversational characteristics of children with semantic-pragmatic disorder. II: What features lead to a judgement of inappropriacy?' *British Journal of Disorders of Communication* **24**(3), 241–63.

Boucher, J. (1998) 'SPD as a distinct diagnostic entity: logical considerations and directions for future research', *International Journal of Language and Communication Disorders* **33**(1), 71–81.

Bradbury, M. (1995) *Rates of Exchange.* Harmondsworth: Penguin.

British Stammering Association (1996) *A Chance to Speak* (videotape). London: British Stammering Association.

Bruner, J. S. (1975) 'The ontogenesis of speech acts', *Journal of Child Language* **2**(1), 1–19.

Butterworth, G. (1998) 'What is special about pointing in babies?' in Simion, F. and Butterworth, G. (eds) *The Development of Sensory, Motor and Cognitive Capacities in Early Infancy*, 171–90. Hove: Psychology Press.

Chomsky, N. (1965) *Aspects of the Theory of Syntax.* Cambridge, MA: MIT Press.

Craig, H. K. (1983) 'Application of pragmatic language models for intervention', in Gallagher, T. M. and Prutting, C. A. (eds) *Pragmatic Assessment and Intervention Issues in Language*, 101–27. San Diego, CA: College-Hill Press, Inc.

Cumine, V. *et al.* (1998) *Asperger Syndrome: A Practical Guide for Teachers.* London: David Fulton Publishers.

Dewart, H. and Summers, S. (1995) *The Pragmatic Profile of Everyday Communication Skills in Children.* Windsor: NFER.

Dockrell, J. E. *et al.* (1998) 'Children with wordfinding difficulties – prevalence, presentation and naming problems', *International Journal of Language and Communication Disorders* **33**(4), 445–54.

Dore, J. (1978) 'Variations in preschool children's conversational performances', in Nelson, K. (ed.) *Children's Language*, 397–444. New York: Gardner Press.

Fawcus, M. (1995) 'Working with adolescents', in Fawcus, M. (ed.) *Stuttering: from Theory to Practice*, 74–98. London: Whurr.

Gallagher, T. M. (ed.) (1991) *Pragmatics of Language: Clinical Practice Issues.* London: Chapman and Hall.

Gleason, J. B. (1985) 'Studying language development', in Gleason, J. B. (ed.) *The Development of Language*, 1–36. Columbus, OH: C. E. Merrill.

Goddard, A. (1997) 'The role of individual educational plans/programmes in special education: a critique', *Support for Learning* **12**(4), 170–74.

Gray, C. (1994a) *Comic Strip Conversations.* Arlington, TX: Future Horizons.

Gray, C. (1994b) *The New Social Stories.* Arlington, TX: Future Horizons.

Gregory, H. and Hill, D. (1984) 'Stuttering therapy for children', in Perkins, W. (ed.) *Stuttering Disorders,* 77–94. New York: Thieme-Stratton.

Grice, H. P. (1981) 'Presupposition and conversational implicature', in Cole, P. (ed.) *Radical Pragmatics,* 183–98. New York: Academic Press.

Guitar, B. (1998) *Stuttering: an Integrated Approach to its Nature and Treatment.* London: Williams and Wilkins.

Halliday, M. A. K. (1975) *Learning How to Mean.* London: Edward Arnold.

Halliday, M. A. K. (1985) *An Introduction to Functional Grammar.* London: Edward Arnold.

Hay, D. F. and Demetriou, H. (1998) 'The developmental origins of social understanding', in Campbell, A. and Muncer, S. (eds) *The Social Child,* 219–48. Hove: Psychology Press.

Hayhow, R. (1995) 'Working with young children', in Fawcus, M. (ed.) *Stuttering: from Theory to Practice,* 44–63. London: Whurr.

Holloway, J. (1994) *A Rainbow of Words.* Stafford: NASEN.

Howlin, P. *et al.* (1999) *Teaching Children with Autism to Mind-read.* Chichester: John Wiley and Sons.

Hsia, H. J. (1977) 'Redundancy: is it the lost key to better communication?' *AV Communication Review* **25**(1), 63–85.

Hyde-Wright, S. (1993) 'Teaching word-finding strategies to severely language-impaired children', *European Journal of Disorders of Communication* **28**(2), 165–75.

Johnson, W. (1942) 'A study of the onset and development of stuttering', *Journal of Speech Disorders* 7(3), 251–57.

Jordan, R. and Powell, S. (1995) *Understanding and Teaching Children with Autism.* Chichester: Wiley.

Kayser, H. (1995) 'Intervention with children from linguistically and culturally diverse backgrounds', in Fey, M. *et al.* (eds) *Language Intervention Preschool through the Elementary Years,* 315–26. Baltimore, MD: Paul H. Brookes.

Kelly, A. (1996) *Talkabout: A Social Communication Skills Package.* Bicester, Oxford: Winslow.

Kelly, E. (1994) 'Speech rates and turn-taking behaviours of children who stutter and their fathers', *Journal of Speech and Hearing Research* 37(6), 1284–94.

Kelly, E. and Conture, E. G. (1992) 'Speaking rates, response time latencies, and interrupting behaviours of young stutterers and their mothers', *Journal of Speech and Hearing Research* 35(6), 1256–67.

Kerbel, D. and Grunwell, P. (1998) 'A study of idiom comprehension in children with semantic-pragmatic difficulties. Part 1: Task effects on the assessment of idiom comprehension in children', *International Journal of Language and Communication Disorders* **33**(1), 1–22.

Kloth, S. *et al.* (1992) 'Communicative style of mothers of incipient stutterers prior to onset'. Paper presented at the American Speech, Language and Hearing Association Annual Convention, San Antonio.

Langlois, A. *et al.* (1986) A comparison of interactions between stuttering children, non-stuttering children and their mothers. *Journal of Fluency Disorders* **11**(3), 263–73.

Lasalle, L. *et al.* (1991) 'Eye-contact between young stutterers and their mothers', *Journal of Fluency Disorders* **16**(2), 173–99.

Lees, R. (1999) 'Stammering children in schools', in McCartney, E. (ed.) *Speech/Language Therapists and Teachers Working Together*, 135–49. London: Whurr.

Legler, D. (1991) *Don't Take it so Literally*. Phoenix, AZ: ECL.

Leicester City Council and Leicestershire County Council (1998) *Asperger Syndrome: Practical Strategies for the Classroom.* London: National Autistic Society.

Leinonen, E. and Kerbel, D. (1999) 'Relevance theory and pragmatic impairment', *International Journal of Language and Communication Disorders* **34**(4), 367–90.

Leinonen, E. and Letts, C. (1997) 'Why pragmatic impairment? A case study in the comprehension of inferential meaning', *European Journal of Disorders of Communication* **35**(2), 35–51.

Leinonen, E. and Smith, B. (1994) 'Appropriacy judgements and pragmatic performance', *European Journal of Disorders of Communication* **29**(1), 77–84.

MacKay, G. F. and Dunn, W. R. (1989) *Early Communicative Skills.* London: Routledge.

MacKay, G. F. and McLarty, M. (1999) 'Pupils with special educational needs', in Bryce, T. G. K. and Humes, W. M. (eds) *Education in Scotland*, 795–804. Edinburgh: Edinburgh University Press.

MacKay, G. F. *et al.* (1996) *Evaluation of the Scottish Centre for Children with Motor Impairments (The Craighalbert Centre): Final Report to the Scottish Office Education Department.* Glasgow: Faculty of Education, University of Strathclyde.

Martin, L. (1990) *Think it, Say it.* Tucson, AZ: Communication Skill Builders.

Mathews, S. *et al.* (1997) 'Parent-child interaction therapy and dysfluency: A single case study', *European Journal of Disorders of Communication* **32**(3), 346–57.

McCartney, E. *et al.* (1998) 'The development of a systems analysis approach to small-scale educational evaluation', *Educational Review* **50**(1), 65–73.

McGregor, K. and Leonard, L. (1995) 'Intervention for word-finding deficits in children', in Fey, M. *et al.* (eds) *Language Intervention Preschool through the Elementary Years*, 85–105. Baltimore, MD: Paul H. Brookes.

McShane, J. (1980) *Learning to Talk.* Cambridge: Cambridge University Press.

McTear, M. and Conti-Ramsden, G. (1992) *Pragmatic Disability in Children.* London: Whurr.

Meyers, S. (1991) 'Interactions with pre-operational preschool stutterers: How will this influence therapy?' in Rustin, L. (ed.) *Parents, Families and the Stuttering Child*, 40–58. Kibworth: Far Communications.

Meyers, S. and Freeman, F. J. (1985) 'Mother and child speech rates as a variable in stuttering and disfluency', *Journal of Speech and Hearing Research* **28**(3), 436–44.

Mosley, J. (1996) *Quality Circle Time in the Primary Classroom.* Wisbech: LDA.

Ninio, A. and Snow, C. E. (1996) *Pragmatic Development.* Oxford: Westview Press.

Ninio, A. *et al.* (1994) 'Classifying communicative acts in children's interactions', *Journal of Communication Disorders* **27**(2), 157–87.

Nippold, M. and Rudzinski, M. (1995) 'Parents' speech and children's stuttering: A critique of the literature', *Journal of Speech and Hearing Research* **38**(5), 978–89.

Park, K. (1995) 'Using objects of reference: A review of the literature', *European Journal of Special Needs Education* **10**(1), 40–6.

Piaget, J. (1952) *The Origins of Intelligence in Children* (Cook, M., trans.). New York: International Universities Press. (Original work published 1936).

Piaget, J. (1954) *The Construction of Reality in the Child* (Cook, M., trans.). New York: Basic Books. (Original work published 1937).

Powell, S. and Jordan, R. (1997) *Autism and Learning: A Guide to Good Practice.* London: David Fulton Publishers.

Prutting, C. A. and Kirchner, D. A. (1983) 'Applied pragmatics', in Gallagher, T. M. and Prutting, C. A. (eds) *Pragmatic Assessment and Intervention Issues in Language*, 28–64. San Diego, CA: College-Hill Press, Inc.

Prutting, C. and Kirchner, D. (1987) 'A clinical appraisal of the pragmatic aspects of language', *Journal of Speech and Hearing Disorders* **52**(1), 105–19.

Rees, N. S. (1978) 'Pragmatics of language', in Schiefelbusch, R. L. (ed.) *Bases of Language Intervention*, 191–268. Baltimore, MD: University Park Press.

Rinaldi, W. (1994) *Social Use of Language Programme.* Windsor: NFER.

Rinaldi, W. (1996) *Understanding Ambiguity: An Assessment of Pragmatic Meaning Comprehension.* Windsor: NFER.

Ross, H. S. and Goldman, B. D. (1977) 'Infants' sociability towards strangers', *Child Development* **48**(2), 638–42.

Rustin, L. (1987) 'The treatment of childhood dysfluency through active parental involvement', in Rustin, L. *et al.* (eds) *Progress in the Treatment of Fluency Disorders*, 166–80. London: Taylor and Francis.

Rustin, L. *et al.* (1995) *The Management of Stuttering in Adolescence.* London: Whurr.

Rustin, L. *et al.* (1996) *Assessment and Therapy for Young Dysfluent Children: Family Interaction.* London: Whurr.

Schulze, H. (1991) 'Time pressure variables in the verbal parent-child interaction patterns of fathers and mothers of stuttering, phonologically disordered and normal preschool children', in Peters, H. *et al.* (eds) *Speech Motor Control and Stuttering*, 441–52. New York: Elsevier Science Publishers.

Schwartz, H. and Conture, E. G. (1988) 'Sub-grouping young stutterers: preliminary behavioural observations', *Journal of Speech and Hearing Research* **31**(1), 62–71.

Searle, J. R. (1969) *Speech Acts: An Essay in the Philosophy of Language.* Cambridge: Cambridge University Press.

Semel, E. *et al.* (1987) *The Clinical Evaluation of Language Fundamentals (Revised).* San Antonio, TX: The Psychological Corporation.

Semel, E. *et al.* (1992) *Clinical Evaluation of Language Fundamentals (Preschool).* San Antonio, TX: The Psychological Corporation.

Smith, J. *et al.* (1997) *Moving Interactions.* San Antonio, TX: Therapy Skill Builders.

Smith, L. (1998) 'Predicting communicative competence at 2 and 3 years from pragmatic skills at 10 months', *International Journal of Language and Communication Disorders* **33**(1), 82–7.

Sperber, D. and Wilson, D. (1995) *Relevance: Communication and Cognition*, 2nd edn. Oxford: Blackwell.

Starkweather, C. W. (1990) 'The demands and capacities model II: clinical applications', *Journal of Fluency Disorders* **15**(2), 143–57.

Stephenson-Opsal, D. and Bernstein Ratner, N. (1988) 'Maternal speech rate modification and childhood stuttering', *Journal of Fluency Disorders* **13**(1), 49–56.

Stern, D. (1977) *The First Relationship: Infant and Mother.* London: Fontana/Open Books.

Stewart, T. and Turnbull, J. (1995) *Working with Dysfluent Children.* Oxford: Winslow.

Thomas, J. (1995) *Meaning in Interaction: An Introduction to Pragmatics.* Harlow: Addison Wesley Longman.

Tough, J. (1976) *Listening to Children Talking.* Cardiff: Drake.

Tough, J. (1977) *The Development of Meaning: A Study of Children's Use of Language.* London: George Allan and Unwin.

Tough, J. (1981) *A Place for Talk.* London: Ward Lock.

Trevarthen, C. (1977) 'Descriptive analyses of infant communicative behaviour', in Schaffer, H. R. (ed.) *Studies in Mother-Infant Interaction,* 227–70. London: Academic Press.

Trevarthen, C. (1988) 'Infants trying to talk: how a child invites communication from the human world', in Söderbergh, R. (ed.) *Children's Creative Communication,* 9–31. Lund: University of Lund Press.

Trevarthen, C. (1993) 'The function of emotions in early infant communication and development', in Nadel, J. and Camaioni, L. (eds) *New Perspectives in Early Communicative Development,* 48–96. London: Routledge.

Trevarthen, C. and Hubley, P. (1978) 'Secondary subjectivity: confidence, confiding and acts of meaning in the first year', in Lock, A. (ed.) *Action, Gesture and Symbol: The Emergence of Language,* 183–229. New York: Academic Press.

Uzgiris, I. C. and Hunt, J, McV. (1975) *Assessment in Infancy.* Champaign, IL: University of Illinois Press.

van Dijk, T. A. (1977) *Text and Context: Explorations in the Semantics and Pragmatics of Discourse.* London: Longman.

Vedelar, L. (1996) 'Pragmatic difficulties and socio-economic problems: a case study', *European Journal of Disorders of Communication* **31**(3), 271–88.

Warden, D. and Christie, D. F. M. (1997) *Teaching Social Behaviour.* London: David Fulton Publishers.

Wing, L. (1996) *The Autistic Spectrum: A Guide for Parents and Professionals.* London: Constable.

Yairi, E. *et al.* (1996) 'Genetics of stuttering: a critical review', *Journal of Speech and Hearing Research* **39**(4), 771–84.

Yaruss, S. J. and Conture, E. G. (1995) 'Mother and child speaking rates and utterance lengths in adjacent fluent utterances: Preliminary observations', *Journal of Fluency Disorders* **20**(3), 257–78.

Zebrowski, P. and Conture, E. G. (1989) 'Judgements of disfluency by mothers of stuttering and normally fluent children', *Journal of Speech and Hearing Research* **32**(3), 625–34.

Zebrowski, P. *et al.* (1996) 'The effect of maternal rate reduction on the stuttering, speech rates and linguistic production of children who stutter: evidence from individual dyads', *Clinical Linguistics and Phonetics* **10**(3), 189–206.

Index